THE GREAT PHYSICIAN'S

Rx *for a*

HEALTHY HEART

JORDAN RUBIN

with Joseph Brasco, MD

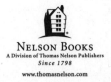

NELSON BOOKS
A Division of Thomas Nelson Publishers
Since 1798

www.thomasnelson.com

All Scripture quotations, unless otherwise indicated, are taken from the NEW KING JAMES VERSION®. Copyright © 1982 by Thomas Nelson, Inc. Used by permission. All right reserved.

Scripture quotations noted NIV are taken from the HOLY BIBLE, NEW INTERNATIONAL VERSION®. Copyright © 1973, 1978, 1984 by International Bible society. Used by permission of Zondervan Bible Publishing House. All right reserved.

Scripture quotations noted NIVare taken from the HOLY BIBLE, NEW INTERNATIONAL VERSION®. Copyright © 1973, 1978, 1984 by International Bible society. Used by permission of Zondervan Bible Publishing House. Use of either trademark requires the permission of International Bible Society.

The "NIV" and "New International Version" trademarks are registered in the United States Patent and Trademark Office by International Bible Society. Use of either trademark requires the permission of International Bible Society.

Scripture quotations noted KJV are from The Holy Bible, KING JAMES VERSION.

Copyright © 2006 by Jordan S. Rubin

All rights reserved. No portion of this book may be reproduced, stored in a retrieval system, or transmitted in any form or by any means—electronic, mechanical, photocopy, recording, scanning, or other—except for brief quotations in critical reviews or articles, without the prior written permission of the publisher.

Published in Nashville, Tennessee, by Thomas Nelson, Inc.

Nelson Books titles may be purchased in bulk for educational, business, fund-raising, or sales promotional use. For information, please e-mail SpecialMarkets@ThomasNelson.com.

Unless otherwise noted, Scripture quotations are taken from the NEW KING JAMES VERSION®. Copyright © 1979, 1980, 1982 by Thomas Nelson, Inc. Used by permission. All rights reserved.

Library of Congress Cataloging-in-Publication Data

Rubin, Jordan.
    The Great Physician's Rx for a healthy heart / by Jordan Rubin with Joseph Brasco.
      p. cm.
    Includes bibliographical references.
    ISBN 0-7852-1433-X (hardcover)
    1. Heart—Diseases—Popular works. 2. Heart—Diseases—Prevention—Popular works.
    3. Heart—Diseases—Religious aspects—Christianity. I. Title: Great Physician's prescription for a healthy heart. II. Brasco, Joseph. III. Title.
RC672.R83 2006
616.1'205—dc22
                                               2006006785

Printed in the United States of America

1 2 3 4 5 6 QW 10 09 08 07 06

To Papa Al and Grandpa Jerry, who left my family and me much too soon, suffering deadly heart attacks at ages fifty-five and sixty-two, respectively. The times we spent together are some of my greatest childhood memories.

CONTENTS

INTRODUCTION

The Heart of the Matter

My son, Joshua, just turned two years old, and in his cute little way, I've found him to be amusing and animated, enthusiastic and emotional—as well as defiant and disobedient on occasion. That makes him a perfectly normal toddler, right?

Joshua is our only child. While my wife, Nicki, and I are sure that we are parents of the most special boy in the entire world, we now have a better understanding of what comedian Bill Cosby meant when he said, "Give me two hundred active two-year-olds, and I can conquer the world." I'm confident Joshua could lead the charge of that army, although the "terrible twos" haven't been too terrible for Nicki and me. That's because we have a better idea of how to handle the little guy after reading the seminal book on disciplining children—*The New Dare to Discipline* by Dr. James Dobson.

Like millions of young parents, we've suddenly discovered that children grow up with wills of their own, which means we need a game plan to raise a healthy, respectful, and happy son. After reading Dr. Dobson's book, we have a better understanding of how to teach Joshua right from wrong and the art of self-control. As our energetic son rambunctiously runs through toddlerhood, Nicki and I are eagerly employing the concepts of reasonable, consistent discipline articulated by Dr. Dobson in his book.

The reason I'm telling you this story is because *The New Dare to Discipline*—a revised and rewritten edition of the 1970 best-selling *Dare to Discipline*—nearly didn't happen. You see, Dr. Dobson suffered a serious heart attack on August 15, 1990, a few months before he was scheduled to begin reworking the bestseller.

A good friend who was a long-time employee of Focus on the Family, the organization founded by Dr. Dobson in the late 1970s, told me that on the morning of August 15, 1990, Dr. Dobson arose early to play pickup basketball at his church, First Church of the Nazarene of Pasadena in Southern California, where his first cousin, H. B. London, was the pastor. The church was home to a nice gym, and Dr. Dobson loved the competition and camaraderie of three-on-three half-court games. A dozen or so friends and staff members of Focus on the Family usually joined him for these early-morning competitions. On this particular summer day in 1990, Dr. Dobson was fifty-four years old, and anyone who watched him play hoops three mornings a week would have pronounced him extremely fit for his age.

Dr. Dobson did not bring his best game to the gym that morning, however. In basketball lingo, he shot bricks at the glass backboard and let players drive by him like his feet were nailed to the polished hardwood floor. After blowing an easy lay-in from underneath the basket, a sharp pain hit Dr. Dobson in the center of his chest. As he caught his breath, he immediately knew something was not right. Perhaps he remembered that this was the same basketball floor where, two years earlier, he had cradled Pistol Pete Maravich in his arms after the forty-year-old basketball legend collapsed and died of a fatal heart attack. When Dr. Dobson's chest pains failed to diminish, he picked up his car keys and waved good-bye. "Sorry, guys, gotta go," he said as he strolled out.

That wasn't like him to quit playing basketball before 8:00 a.m. One of the players ran after Dr. Dobson, asking him if he was feeling all right. "I think I'm okay," he said, but something told him that he wasn't 100 percent.

Instead of going home to shower, Dr. Dobson drove himself to a nearby hospital, St. Luke's of Pasadena, where he parked the car and gathered his thoughts. To march into an emergency room and announce that he was experiencing chest pains would blow a huge hole in his hyper-busy schedule: meetings with the executive staff, broadcast tapings, and responding to the dozens of phone messages fielded by his personal assistants. He prided himself on keeping up with "the stack"—a foot-high mountain of memos and correspondence that came his way in those days before e-mail. He also realized—from his days of being part of the University of Southern California medical school faculty—that walking into a hospital and saying, "I think I'm having a heart attack," would commit him to three days of tests and medical observation.

Dr. Dobson sat in his car for nearly thirty minutes, weighing the consequences of stepping through the emergency room doors. "What do You want me to do, Lord?" he prayed. "I'm fifty-four years old, and I'm having chest pains."

It's a good thing Dr. Dobson admitted himself at St. Luke's that morning, because tests revealed that he had suffered a mild-to-moderate heart attack. Apparently, one of the five coronary arteries supplying the heart with blood became blocked. Thanks to quick intervention, Dr. Dobson received the medical care he needed to stay alive. In many ways, Dr. Dobson was a fortunate man because his cardiologist determined that several collateral arteries compensated for the closed artery, which prevented permanent damage—or death—from occurring. Those collateral arteries had developed from the vigorous basketball games over the years.

Still, it was a close call for Dr. Dobson, who had plenty of time for reflection during his ten-day hospital stay. He certainly thought about how close he had been to dying just like his father, James Dobson Sr., who succumbed to a heart attack thirteen years earlier. His sixty-six-year-old father died in December 1977 when his heart gave out, just seventy-one days after surviving his first heart attack. On the air and in his writings, Dr. Dobson called his father his greatest friend, his most trusted advisor, and the person who led a son to choose his values, his dreams, and his God.

Was he destined to die early as well? For Dr. Dobson, a heart attack in his mid-fifties was more than the proverbial wake-up call: it prompted the Focus on the Family founder to undergo major lifestyle changes, especially in what he ate.

SWEEPING CHANGES

A young James Dobson was raised on the standard meat-and-potatoes, pass-the-bread-please, all-American diet of the 1950s.

Born in Shreveport, Louisiana, his family hopped around before settling in San Benito, Texas, during his high school years. Meanwhile, he learned to enjoy the staples of good eatin' in the South: fried chicken, mashed potatoes swimming in gravy, country-fried steak, and apple pie à la mode. After attending college in the Southern California area, he married Shirley and finished his doctorate at the University of Southern California. There, he fell into a routine: breakfast was two doughnuts and two cups of coffee, lunch was a chili burger and fries; dinner was whatever, and there was always room for dessert at Baskin-Robbins, where he ordered a hot fudge sundae or toffee ice cream every night.

During this time, Dr. Dobson developed a fondness for Tommy's, a red-roofed A-frame burger joint whose claim to fast-food fame centered around a six-inch-high temple of grease known as the Chili Burger: two beef patties smothered with chili, fresh-chopped onions, a slice of beefsteak tomato, and double-thick American cheese. Sure, a single Tommy's Chili Burger contained 490 calories and twenty-two grams of fat, but who was searching out nutritional facts in those days?

Following his heart attack, however, the lunchtime forays to Tommy's were over. So were delicious fried-food meals topped off with icky-sweet desserts. Dr. Dobson totally revamped his diet: he only ate grilled chicken or fish (and no red meat), fresh garden salads, plenty of fruits and vegetables, and no fried foods, no white bread, and nothing with sugar, butter, or sour cream. He joked on his radio broadcast that he was destined to eat "birdseed" the rest of his life.

Dr. Dobson also kicked up his fitness level a notch. Since quick-moving basketball was judged to be too strenuous on his heart, he brought a treadmill into his home and walked briskly for an hour while catching up on the morning news shows before his departure to the Focus on the Family campus. He took exercise so seriously that he never missed a day for years at a time.

Since his heart attack in 1990, Dr. Dobson has done a lot more than revise *Dare to Discipline*. In the last sixteen years, he's probably recorded 1,500 radio programs, written or revised a dozen books, appeared scores of times on shows like *Larry King Live* and *Hannity & Colmes*, and spoken up about pro-family issues with the movers and shakers in Washington, D.C.—all because he survived a grim encounter with the "silent killer"—a stoppage of blood flow to the heart. He knew he was fortunate to be alive; Dr. Dobson declared in his monthly newsletter that "about a million prayers saved my life."

Statistically speaking, Dr. Dobson needed divine intervention to survive his heart attack. Of the estimated 700,000 Americans who are hit with a sudden coronary attack each year, an estimated 180,000 will not survive.[1] Heart attacks and other cardiovascular diseases (CVD) are this country's number-one cause of death, according to the American Heart Association's latest compilation of "Heart Disease and Stroke Statistics."[2] A total of 910,614 Americans died from various cardiovascular diseases in 2003, the most recent year that data was available at time of this printing.[3] Cardiovascular diseases include high blood pressure, coronary heart disease (heart attacks and angina), congestive heart failure, strokes, and congenital heart defects.

The public perception of a heart attack is *boom!*—you're gone. Perhaps that's from viewing *The Godfather* on DVD too often and watching Don Corleone keel over in his tomato bushes to meet his Maker and escape retribution from New York's other crime bosses. That's par for the course in Hollywood, where it seems that the protagonist suffering a heart attack clutches his chest, rolls his eyes, slumps into unconsciousness, and takes his final breath within seconds of hitting the ground.

If you've noticed that I'm referring to men here, then allow me to ask this question: When was the last time you saw a woman suffer a dramatic heart attack on the silver screen or the Lifetime Channel? You never see women die of a heart attack in Hollywood, although women account for nearly half of all heart-attack deaths, and one-third of all women die from some form of heart disease.[4]

Whether you're male or female, the truth is that two-thirds of heart-attack victims don't keel over and die like in the movies. More often than not, a deadly heart attack is preceded months, days, and hours by episodes of chest pain, shortness of breath, and a tingly sensation in the left arm. Others feel a sharp pain to the chest, as Dr. Dobson did, or nausea, pain radiating to the neck and arms, and cold, clammy skin.

The medical term for heart attack is myocardial infarction, which sounds like something Will Ferrell would say to get a cheap laugh. There's nothing funny, though, about a myocardial infarction, because doctors estimate that you have a five-minute survivability window to call 911 and get paramedics on the scene. This polysyllabic phrase is derived from three Latin roots:

myo, meaning muscle; *cardial,* meaning heart; and *infarction,* meaning the death of tissue due to a lack of blood supply.

The heart is probably the most amazing organ that God created. Beating in a stable rhythm for sixty, seventy, or more times per minute—more than one hundred thousand times per day— the heart sends a steady supply of blood to the body's muscles and organs without skipping a beat. This fist-sized muscle is actually two pumps in one: the right side of the heart receives blood from the body and pumps it into the lungs; the left side of the heart receives blood from the lungs and pumps these oxygen-rich nutrients to the furthest reaches of the body twenty-four hours a day, seven days a week.

Cardiovascular problems begin cropping up when the coronary arteries carrying blood away from the heart plug up with fatty matter, or plaque. The plaque deposits, which are hard on the outside but soft and mushy on the inside, attract blood components, which stick to the artery wall lining. This fatty buildup can break open and form a blood clot, reducing or blocking blood flow. When blood flow is reduced by a small amount, you feel chest pain, also known as angina. When a blood clot suddenly cuts off all or most of the blood supply, the heart muscle is starved for oxygen. Within a short time, the death of heart muscle cells occurs—the official start of a myocardial infarction, or heart attack.

Sometimes death is instantaneous, as was the case with Pistol Pete Maravich, and other times it's survivable, as Dr. Dobson happily found out. The amount of damage to the heart depends on the size of the area supplied by the blocked artery and the passage of time from the onset of symptoms to prompt medical care.

CONVENTIONAL TREATMENT

When paramedics and EMTs respond to a 911 call, they know they are racing against the clock. If your heart stops pumping and you stop breathing, irreversible brain damage starts within four to six minutes. Paramedics usually employ a defibrillator to resuscitate heart-attack victims. They attach a pair of paddles to the heart area, sending electrical shock waves to stimulate the heart to resume beating.

Once you're stabilized, you're rushed to the hospital, where ER doctors immediately spring into action. In quick order, they introduce drugs to dissolve blood clots and often perform an emergency angioplasty—a procedure in which doctors position a catheter inside the clogged arteries and employ a small balloon to clear away the blockage. The faster doctors can perform this Roto-Rooter action, the greater the patient's chance of survival. The entire process, which is known as reperfusion, can be done in less than an hour and sometimes as quickly as thirty minutes.

But let's say that you're like Dr. Dobson, experiencing the classic symptoms of a heart attack: chest pains, shortness of breath, a prolonged crushing pressure in the center of the chest, or tingling in the arms. You feel ill enough to call 911 or your family doctor.

Like Dr. Dobson, once you mention that you're having chest pains to a medical professional, you'll be making an unscheduled trip to a hospital emergency room, where doctors will run a battery of tests, including the following:

- An electrocardiogram, or EKG, which checks the heart's rhythm and can locate the area where the heart attack could be occurring

- Various blood tests, including the search for substances in the blood called biomarkers, which tell your doctors if heart cells have been injured

- Stress tests, which pinpoint blockages in blood vessels

- Computed tomography (CT or CAT) scans, which are diagnostic imaging procedures that use X-ray and computer technology to allow doctors to view the damaged areas of the heart, including problems with the heart's ability to pump blood to the body

Following the comprehensive testing, doctors review the results. They may choose to prescribe certain medications to break up or prevent blood clots and prevent platelets from gathering and sticking to the plaque. Or doctors may say that you're a strong candidate for the aforementioned angioplasty or coronary artery bypass surgery, the most commonly performed heart operation all over the world, with more than three hundred thousand procedures performed in the United States every year. In this procedure, surgeons use a vein (usually taken from the patient's leg) or synthetic arterial-like material to connect the aorta on one end to the coronary artery beyond the area of obstruction. In the U.S., these surgeries generally cost more than twenty thousand dollars.

Critics point out that coronary bypass surgery consumes more of our medical dollars than any other treatment or procedure. Coronary artery bypass surgery is "the leader in terms of equipment and personnel, hospital space, and total associated revenues," points out Thomas A. Preston, MD, chief of cardiology at the Pacific Medical Center in Seattle. "The operation is heralded by the popular press, aggrandized by the medical profession, and actively sought by the consuming public."[5]

Not all those suffering from cardiovascular disease are destined to go under the knife, however. The conventional playbook for fighting heart disease without invasive surgery involves treating high blood pressure or lowering cholesterol with medications. Heart-attack survivors are routinely given aspirin, which reduces the tendency of platelets in the blood to clump and clot. Other "medication therapies" include: nitroglycerin, which relaxes the muscular wall of the blood vessels; ACE (angiotensin converting enzyme) inhibitors such as Vasotec, Zestril, and Prinvil, which reduce the stress load on the heart; and beta-blocking agents that reduce the risk of future heart attacks. When you've regained your strength—and doctors are confident that you're not a candidate for a recurrent heart attack—they send you home with instructions to take it easy, which is always easier said than done.

Heart bypass surgery, angioplasty procedures, and cholesterol-lowering drugs have become major industries in this country since the United States leads the world in death rates from heart disease. Today, it's estimated that more than sixty million Americans—around one-fourth of the adult population—suffer from some form of cardiovascular disease. Dr. Preston has a point: the medical bill to treat heart disease and strokes in 2005 was $395 billion, according to the American Heart Association and National Heart, Lung, and Blood Institute. It must always be said that the cost of physicians, hospital and nursing home services, medications, and other medical durables do not compare to the emotional cost of human suffering and lost lives that cardiovascular disease inflicts upon individuals and families.

ALTERNATIVE TREATMENTS

One of the most popular alternatives to conventional angioplasty and coronary bypass surgery is chelation (pronounced ke-LA-shun) therapy, in which the organic chemical ethylenediaminetetraacetic acid (EDTA) is introduced either intravenously or in supplement form into the body to remove plaque and calcium deposits attached to the arterial walls. The offending material is then excreted through the body's urine.

The main organization promoting chelation therapy is the American College for Advancement in Medicine (ACAM), which claims that the therapy is effective against atherosclerosis, coronary heart disease, and peripheral vascular disease. My friend Garry Gordon, MD, D.O. (Doctor of Osteopathy), considered to be the father of modern EDTA chelation therapy, said, "Let's look at a group of my patients with any level of stageable disease and simply see how many of them are alive at the end of five years, compared with those on any other standard therapy. I couldn't believe it when I went to the meetings with the big cardiologists and found that they consider the diagnosis of congestive heart failure to be virtually a death sentence, because over 60 percent of their patients are dead within the first year. I haven't lost one patient with congestive heart failure in ten years! It shocks me how big a difference there is, depending on which school of medicine you follow."[6]

The American Heart Association, however, has found no scientific evidence demonstrating any benefit from this form of therapy. "Up to now, there have been no adequate, controlled, published scientific studies using currently approved scientific methodology to support this therapy for cardiovascular disease," said an American Heart Association press release. "The United States Food and Drug Administration (FDA), the National Institutes of Health (NIH) and the American College of Cardiology all agree with the American Heart Association on this point."[7]

Another alternative treatment for heart disease is hyperbaric oxygen therapy (HBOT), which some in the medical profession believe deserves consideration. Proponents say that placing patients in a hyperbaric chamber cuts in half the time required for the heart to resume normal electrical activity and raises the "ejection faction"—the heart's ability to pump blood. In hyperbaric therapy, a patient lies on a padded table that slides into a clear plastic tube that is seven feet long. The chamber is gradually pressurized with pure oxygen until it reaches twice the normal atmospheric pressure. Patients, who are reminded to relax and breathe normally during treatment, may experience ear popping or mild discomfort, which usually disappears if the pressure is lowered a bit.

Hyperbaric oxygen therapy has yet to become standard equipment in ER bays because of the cost of each chamber (over $100,000) and the medical establishment's lack of confidence as to its efficacy. The Food and Drug Administration has approved only thirteen uses for hyperbaric oxygen therapy, and cardiovascular diseases and heart attacks are not on that list.

A ROAD MAP FROM HERE

Do lifestyle factors increase or decrease the risk of coronary heart disease and heart attack? The American Heart Association says their significance and prevalence haven't been precisely determined, which I can accept, but I'm sure few in the medical establishment would disagree with the following statement: *You take care of your heart, and your heart will take care of you.*

Yes, genetics can play a role, and about one out of every 125 infants is born with heart defects each year in the United States.[8] For them, their hearts are like ticking time bombs until suddenly they stop . . . ticking . . . as was the case with Pete Maravich, who was born with a rare congenital defect—one coronary artery system instead of two. Following his sudden death, astounded doctors wondered how he lived so many years playing such a demanding sport.

But if you're eating like a pig, drinking like a fish, and smoking like a chimney—to rattle off three clichés—then you're just as much a walking time bomb as poor Pistol Pete was. If your idea of exercise is walking into a McDonald's instead of driving through the drive-thru window, then I would make sure your life insurance is paid up, because each year, each month, and each morning is a roll of the dice.

I believe cardiovascular disease—except for those born with a genetic defect, of course—is highly preventable for those who follow *The Great Physician's Rx for a Healthy Heart.* My approach is based on 7 Keys to unlock the body's healthy potential that were established in my foundational book, *The Great Physician's Rx for Health and Wellness.* The 7 Keys are:

- Key #1: Eat to Live

- Key #2: Supplement Your Diet with Whole Food Nutritionals, Living Nutrients, and Superfoods

- Key #3: Practice Advanced Hygiene

- Key #4: Condition Your Body with Exercise and Body Therapies

- Key #5: Reduce Toxins in Your Environment

- Key #6: Avoid Deadly Emotions

- Key #7: Live a Life of Prayer and Purpose

Since you're reading this book, I figure that you probably know something about cardiovascular disease or heart attacks, either from personal experience or because a spouse or family member recently survived one or—even worse—didn't. If so, please know that I'm writing *The Great Physician's Rx for a Healthy Heart* for you. Whether you've contemplated your mortality or watched a loved one try to bounce back from a life-threatening heart attack, you're motivated to do something. You understand that this is the disease of second chances: surviving a heart attack is like being given another opportunity to ride the merry-go-round of life. If that's the case, I welcome you to *The Great Physician's Rx for a Healthy Heart*.

A healthy heart pumps life-sustaining nutrients throughout the body, supplying you with the energy you need to attack the day, be there for your kids, and fulfill God's purpose for your life. It's been said that you change your life by changing your heart. Do you need a change of heart before you can wholeheartedly adopt the Great Physician's Rx for a healthy heart in your life?

Please understand that *The Great Physician's Rx for a Healthy Heart* is not guaranteed to prevent or treat cardiovascular disease, and I would never want anyone to represent this book as promising a "cure" to this deadly malady. My great hope is that the 7 Keys will do one of two things for you:

1. Give you the best possible chance to live a long, healthy life without ever developing cardiovascular disease.

2. Augment whatever therapy—conventional or alternative—you're seeking to treat your heart disease.

In closing, I'm glad Dr. Dobson survived so that Nicki and I could be the beneficiaries of his child-rearing advice. I'm pleased to hear that he overhauled his diet and made a daily workout on the treadmill a priority—actions that are part of the Great Physician's Rx for health and wellness. God obviously had a plan to keep using Dr. Dobson, just as He has a plan to use you.

But for that to happen, He needs you at your physical, spiritual, and emotional best.

KEY #1

Eat to Live

When someone suffers a heart attack in midlife, as Dr. Dobson did, doctors often put the fear of God into them when it comes to their diet.

Lay off the Ruth's Chris steaks.
No more deep-dish, double-crust pizza.
Shake your salt habit.
Get rid of butter.
And no nuts.

The conventional wisdom among the medical establishment these days is that a high-cholesterol diet promotes coronary heart disease, and from my reading, this article of faith is one of the most deeply ingrained beliefs in modern medicine. Cardiologists point to the Framingham Heart Study, which began in 1948 when researchers recruited 5,209 men and women between the ages of thirty and sixty-two from the town of Framingham, Massachusetts, and began the first round of extensive physical examinations and lifestyle interviews that would be analyzed for common patterns related to cardiovascular disease development.[1]

Over the last five decades, the detailed medical histories, physical examinations, and laboratory tests on the study volunteers have reputedly established high blood cholesterol as a major risk factor for coronary heart disease. The comprehensive study, conducted by the National Heart Institute (now known as the National Heart, Lung, and Blood Institute, or NHLBI) concluded that cholesterol hardens arteries carrying vital oxygen and nutrients to and from the heart.

The Framingham Heart Study spurred the drug industry to develop statin drugs that would interrupt the formation of cholesterol inside the body. Statins are a class of drugs used to lower blood cholesterol, and these pills prompt the liver to block a substance the body needs to produce cholesterol while helping the body reabsorb cholesterol that has accumulated in plaques clinging to the arterial walls. Commonly prescribed statins include:

- Lipitor (atorvastatin)
- Pravachol (pravastatin)
- Lescol (fluvastatin)
- Mevacor (lovastatin)
- Crestor (rosuvastatin calcium)
- Zocor (simvastatin)

I would imagine that you recognize the first statin drug on this list: Lipitor. Racking up $11 billion in sales in 2005, Lipitor is the best-selling drug in the world and a cash cow for Pfizer, the makers of Viagra. If you happen to be forty years of age or older (and especially a male), submit to an annual physical, have blood drawn, and learn that you have a total cholesterol level higher than two hundred, your family physician will likely write you a prescription for Lipitor. It's practically automatic these days and one reason why 12 million Americans, or 4 percent of the U.S. population, are swallowing this cholesterol-lowering drug with their morning OJ despite its cost: most pay around seven to eight hundred dollars a year for their Lipitor.[2]

Lipitor and its statin cousins are potent medicines that usually reduce cholesterol levels, but not without extracting a cost. So-called "minor" side effects are nausea, diarrhea, constipation, and muscle aches. Two potentially serious side effects are elevated liver enzymes (medicalese for liver damage) and statin myopathy (kidney failure), and the long-term side effects are not known at this time.

I'm convinced, though, that if you eat the foods that are part of *The Great Physician's Rx for a Healthy Heart*, you may make a visit to your physician, have him or her take a blood test, and find that your cholesterol is within the normal range. Then you can flush those expensive cholesterol-reducing drugs down the toilet (as long as you and your doctor are agreed on that course of action, of course).

Our bodies do need cholesterol, a soft, waxlike substance produced by the liver and found in the bloodstream and all the body's cells. Cholesterol digests fats, is the source material for cell membranes and various hormones, and serves other much-needed bodily functions. While the liver makes around 1,000 milligrams of cholesterol daily, the body receives an additional 200 to 500 milligrams of cholesterol from foods such as meats, poultry, fish, eggs, butter, cheese, and whole milk. Fruits, vegetables, and cereals do not have cholesterol.

Cholesterol is transported in the bloodstream by lipoproteins—

actually, two different ones. A high-density lipoprotein (HDL) is known as the "good cholesterol" because it collects unused cholesterol and transports it back to the liver, where it is destroyed. A low-density lipoprotein (LDL) is public enemy number one, however, because this "bad cholesterol" builds up and clings to the inside of the arteries. Medical researchers have learned that large numbers of LDL particles are strongly associated with coronary heart disease. Thus, physicians pay close attention to LDL numbers, and there's a push in modern medicine to drive LDL levels below 100 milligrams per deciliter (mg/dl) for men and 110 mg/dl for women through the use of statin drugs like Lipitor or Pravachol.

Lately, however, I've encountered a push back in certain medical circles, and the charge is being led by a Swedish physician, Dr. Uffe Ravnskov, who earned his Ph.D. for his scientific studies at the Departments of Nephrology and Clinical Chemistry at the University Hospital in Lund, Sweden.

Dr. Ravnskov followed the scientific literature about cholesterol and cardiovascular disease for years, and throughout that time, he could never recall a study showing that high cholesterol was dangerous to the heart or the coronary arteries. Yet the medical grapevine around the world was heavily influenced by the Framingham Heart Study, which pointed the finger at cholesterol as the culprit for the leading cause of death in the United States.

From Dr. Ravnskov's viewpoint, however, the emperor—King Cholesterol—wore no clothes, because as best as he could tell, medical studies did not conclusively prove the connection between high cholesterol levels and cardiovascular disease. The Swedish doctor wrote nearly forty medical papers critical of the alleged association between cholesterol and cardiovascular disease.

For instance, he pointed out that in a thirty-year follow-up of the Framingham population, high cholesterol wasn't predictive for a heart attack after the age of forty-seven, and those whose cholesterol went down had the biggest risk of having a heart attack! His citation came straight from the Framingham study: "For each 1 mg/dl drop of cholesterol, there was an 11 percent *increase* in coronary and total mortality" (emphasis added).[3]

Pointing out inconsistencies earned Dr. Ravnskov a reputation in the cardiology community as a gadfly at best and a bomb thrower at worst. His critical but scientific analysis was of little interest to the editors of the *Journal of American Medicine* (*JAMA*) or the *New England Journal of Medicine* (*NEJM*), nor to the mainstream medical community, which continued to advise patients to limit their intake of fats, including those rich in saturated fatty acids, to reduce their risk of dying from cardiovascular disease.

Stymied in his attempts to find an audience among his peers, Dr. Ravnskov put down his concerns in a book called *The Cholesterol Myths*, first published in Sweden in 1991—in Swedish. The book was largely ignored and produced little impact. Even worse, critics on a Finnish TV show burned his book on the air! Several years passed, and Dr. Ravnskov thought that having *The Cholesterol Myths* published in English would jump-start the discussion. Queries to literary agents and publishers in Great Britain and the United States were summarily rejected, however.

Then the Internet arrived on the scene in the latter half of the 1990s. Suddenly, Dr. Ravnskov didn't need a publisher; he posted a few chapters of *The Cholesterol Myths* on the Web, and presto, he was no longer a pariah tilting against windmills, fighting a lost cause like Don Quixote. As word of mouth built—and people typed in "cholesterol and heart disease" in their search engines—Dr. Ravnskov received e-mails from those impressed with his measured and clear-eyed analysis, including researchers skeptical about the "diet-heart" connection percolating through the medical community.

Dr. Ravnskov's work confirms my belief that the oft-recommended low-fat, low-cholesterol diet touted for preventing heart disease will never be the hoped-for panacea. Too many doctors are recommending that people not eat certain foods that can actually be quite beneficial to heart health.

I'm getting ahead of myself here, but certain "high fat" foods—steak, eggs, butter, and dairy products, when consumed from free-range and organic sources—contain fats that your body needs for optimal health. God, in His infinite wisdom, created certain fats to do the following functions: play a vital role in bone health, enhance the immune system, protect the liver from alcohol and other toxins, and guard against harmful microorganisms in the digestive tract.

The best examples of "good fats" are healthy saturated fats, omega-3 polyunsaturated fats, and monounsaturated (omega-9) fatty acids. You can find these fats in a wide range of foods, including salmon, lamb, and goat meat, goat's and sheep's milk and cheese, coconut, walnuts, olives, almonds, and avocados. These fats provide us with a concentrated source of energy and are the source material for cell membranes and various hormones.

Ah, you may ask, "Didn't the Creator know that fats and cholesterol are the main causes of coronary disease?"

Yes, He did, but it's the foods with *trans fats* that most likely are at the root of our national epidemic of cardiovascular disease. Trans fats are artery-clogging fats produced by heating liquid vegetable oils in the presence of hydrogen to make them solid at room temperature—a process known as hydrogenation. Food conglomerates routinely utilize hydrogenated oil in their manufacturing plants, which means that trans fats are found in nearly all our processed foods—foods that God definitely did *not* create.

I'm talking about vegetable shortening, frozen pizza, ice cream, processed cheese, potato chips, cookie dough, white bread, dinner rolls, snack foods, doughnuts, candy, salad dressing, margarine—the list is endless. Why do food producers employ so much chemistry? Because it allows them to produce a more competitively priced product with a longer shelf life. Commercially prepared fried foods, like French fries and onion rings fried in polyunsaturated vegetable oils, also contain gobs of trans fat.

One big problem with trans fat is the number it does on your cholesterol levels. Consumption of foods with trans fat raises your bad LDL and lowers the good HDL, which elevates the risk of heart disease as well as type 2 diabetes. Scientists have been warning us for years that eating trans fat can lead to heart problems, which is why in 2006 the U.S. Food and Drug

Administration began requiring companies to state the amount of trans fat as part of the nutrition facts.

LAYING THE GROUNDWORK

My first key—"Eat to Live"—happens to be the most important prescription in *The Great Physician's Rx for a Healthy Heart*, because what you choose to nourish yourself with will either positively or negatively affect the health of your heart—your most important muscle—as well as your entire body. The best way to "eat to live" can be summed up by these two foundational principles:

1. Eat what God created for food.

2. Eat food in a form that is healthy for the body.

Eating food that God created in a form that is healthy for the body means choosing foods as close to the natural source as possible, which will nourish your body, help your heart beat strong and continuous, and give you the healthiest life possible. As you have probably figured out by now, I'm a proponent of natural foods grown organically since these are foods that God created in a form healthy for the body.

Optimizing nutrition begins with an awareness of what you are sending to your digestive tract. To begin with, everything you put into your mouth is a protein, a fat, or a carbohydrate. Let's take a closer look at these macronutrients:

THE FIRST WORD ON PROTEINS

Proteins, one of the basic components of foods, are the essential building blocks of the body and involved in the function of every living cell. One of proteins' main tasks is to provide specific nutrient material to grow and repair cells—especially the heart muscle. Researchers at the University of Texas Southwestern Medical Center in Dallas are studying how a protein named thymosin beta-4 protects the heart muscle from damage and even triggers the repair of the heart following a coronary attack.[4]

All proteins are combinations of twenty-two amino acids, which build and maintain the body's organs, including the heart, as well as the muscles and nerves, to name a few important duties. Your body, however, cannot produce all twenty-two amino acids that you need to live a robust life. Scientists have discovered that eight essential amino acids are missing, meaning that they must come from sources outside the body. I know the following fact drives vegetarians and vegans crazy, but animal protein—chicken, beef, lamb, dairy, eggs, etc.—is the *only* complete protein source providing the Big Eight amino acids in the right quantities and ratios.

The best approach for a healthy heart is eating the leanest, healthiest sources of animal protein available, which come from organically raised cattle, sheep, goats, buffalo, and deer—animals that graze on pastureland grasses. Lean grass-fed beef is lower in calories and doesn't contain as much fat as grain-fed beef.

I'm also a huge fan of free-range chicken and eating fish captured from lakes, streambeds, or ocean depths. Fish with scales and fins caught in the wild are excellent sources of protein, as well as healthy fats, vitamins, and minerals, and they provide all the essential amino acids. Wild fish, which is nutritionally far superior to farm raised, should be consumed liberally.

A REPRISE ON FATS

I've already mentioned how trans fat clogs arteries like sludge in a drainpipe. Yet eating healthy fats can have a protective effect against heart disease. I'm referring to foods loaded with the following:

- polyunsaturated fats (high in omega-3 fatty acids)
- monounsaturated (omega-9) fatty acids
- conjugated linoleic acid (CLA)
- key omega-6 fats such as GLA
- healthy saturated fats containing short- and medium-chain fatty acids, such as butter and coconut oil

These good fats are found in a wide range of foods, including salmon, cod liver oil, lamb and goat meat, high omega-3 eggs, flaxseeds, walnuts, olives, macadamia nuts, avocados, butter from grass-fed animals, and dairy products derived from goat's milk, sheep's milk, and cow's milk.

The problem with the standard American diet is that people

eat too many of the wrong foods containing the wrong fats and not enough of the right foods with the right fats. Two of the top fats and oils on my list are extra virgin coconut and olive oils, which are beneficial to the body and aid metabolism. I urge you to cook with extra virgin coconut oil, which is an extremely healthy food that few people have ever heard of.

GO FOR THOSE CARBS

By definition, carbohydrates are the starches and sugars produced by plant foods, and they are carried in the blood as glucose and regulated by insulin, a hormone that holds the key to each cell's nutritional door. Thanks to the low-carb diet popularized by two cardiologists—Dr. Robert Atkins and Dr. Arthur Agatston—creators of the Atkins diet and the South Beach diet, respectively, Americans have been on a carbohydrate witch hunt for the last decade or so. Low-carb diets are touted as a good regime for heart patients, especially those who need to lose weight.

The Atkins diet, to single out the oldest and most widely practiced modern-day, low-carb diet, calls for a high consumption of conventionally raised and processed meats (ham, bacon, pepperoni, salami, and hot dogs) that are high in unhealthy fats, which can only increase your risk of a heart attack. The Atkins diet also forbids plentiful amounts of fruits and high-starch vegetables, which are loaded with fiber and antioxidant and thus are heart-healthy.

So I have a question: How does one reconcile that nutritional advice with the American Heart Association recommendation that we eat at least five servings of fruits and vegetables daily to significantly reduce three of the major risk factors for a heart attack—high blood cholesterol, high blood pressure, and excess body weight? The American Heart Association also recommends skinless poultry and lean meats.

If you're recovering from a heart attack, I don't believe you need to curb your carbs. Instead, you should add unrefined carbohydrates including the aforementioned fruits and veggies as well as whole grains such as oats, wheat, rye, corn, rice, and barley to your diet. Unrefined carbohydrates contain the whole grain, including the bran and the germ, so they're higher in fiber and the healthy fatty acids.

One of the best unrefined carbohydrates for heart health is whole oats, which contain beta-glucans from soluble fiber. The U.S. Food and Drug Administration concluded that there is a link between the soluble fiber in whole-oat foods and a reduction in coronary heart disease risk because the beta-glucan soluble fiber is the primary component responsible for lowering the bad LDL cholesterol levels.[5] That's why you're seeing a lot more red hearts on cereal boxes like Quaker Oats oatmeal and Kashi Heart to Heart cereal.

Unfortunately, much of the cereal—and bread—in this country is made from wheat and other grains subjected to an "enriching" process. The only thing enriched flour "enriches" is the bad LDL cholesterol levels, perhaps triglycerides in the blood, and, of course, insulin levels, which is why foods made with enriched flour should be avoided completely, especially if you're recovering from a heart attack. Instead, buy organic flour with the words "stone ground," "yeast free," or "sprouted" on the package label. These whole grain products—along with "old-fashioned" oatmeal—haven't been stripped of their vital fiber, vitamin, and mineral components. The Harvard School of Public Health analyzed diet and health records of more than twenty-seven thousand men ages forty to seventy-five over a period of fourteen years and found that those eating the most whole grains cut their heart-disease risk by almost 20 percent.[6]

When folks have heart problems, they often think that they have to curtail their carbs, but consuming carbohydrates that are low glycemic, high nutrient, and low sugar are heart friendly. I'm talking about most high-fiber fruits (such as berries), vegetables, nuts, seeds, legumes, cultured dairy products, and grains.

Eating foods high in fiber will immediately improve your blood sugar levels by slowing the absorption of sugars into your bloodstream. A diet high in fiber can reduce a woman's risk of coronary heart disease by up to 23 percent, according to a study released in the *Journal of the American Medical Association*. After controlling for various factors, researchers found that women who consumed the most fiber each day, around twenty-three grams, reduced their risk of coronary heart disease.[7]

The Great Physician's Nutritional Recommendations

Following a heart attack, most doctors and nurses will stress the importance of fruits, vegetables, whole grain breads and cereals, moderate amounts of meat and dairy products, and cutting back on sugar and fats.

While I concur with much of what conventional medicine recommends for cardiovascular patients regarding their nutrition, I want to make some additional points about the staples of most diets, as well as offer my own recommendations.

First, let me remind you to chew your food well. If people tease you about "inhaling" your food, then you're eating too fast. I recommend chewing each mouthful of food twenty-five to seventy-five times before swallowing. This advice may sound ridiculous, but I know that a conscious effort to chew food slowly ensures that plenty of digestive juices are added to the food as it begins to wind through the digestive tract.

Got enough to chew on? Good. Let's take a closer look at what you should and shouldn't be eating when it comes to having a healthy heart:

1. Meats

Conventional wisdom among the cardiovascular community is that heart attack victims should reduce their consumption of red meat, which contains more saturated fat and cholesterol than fish or white poultry meat. The American Heart Association recommends eating no more than six ounces of cooked lean meat, poultry, or fish a day. Lean beef cuts are round, chuck, sirloin, or loin.

A lot has been written about the dangers of meat—especially beef—causing heart disease. Yes, if you eat assembly-line cuts of flank steak from hormone-injected cattle eating pesticide-sprayed feed laced with antibiotics, this could pose a problem for your heart. A much better solution would be eating meat from organically raised cattle, sheep, goats, buffalo, and venison that graze on nature's bountiful grasses.

Grass-fed meats and fish caught in the wild are high in vitamins B_{12} and B_6, which is significant information in regards to cardiovascular disease. In recent years, researchers have identified another risk factor for cardiovascular disease known as an elevated homocysteine level. Homocysteine, an amino acid, is normally found in blood, but elevated levels impair endothelial vasomotor function, which is medicalese for how easily blood flows through blood vessels. High levels of homocysteine damage coronary arteries and make it easier for blood-clotting cells called platelets to clump together and form a clot. Blood clots are a precursor to heart attacks.[8]

Since vitamins B_{12} and B_6 are involved in homocysteine metabolism, eating grass-fed beef and wild-caught fish cause a decrease in homocysteine levels in the blood, which is good for the heart. Wild trout, for example, is one of the highest sources of natural B_{12}, along with salmon and sockeye.

Just as there are meats you should eat for your heart health, there are certain meats you must avoid. I'm talking about breakfast links, bacon, lunch meats, ham, hot dogs, bratwurst, and other sausages. These meats use preservatives called nitrates to give meats their blood-red color, convey flavor, and resist the development of botulism spores. Nitrates can convert to nitrites, and nitrites have been studied for decades in public and private settings for their ability to cause cancer and tumors in test animals.

I have other reasons for recommending that you stay away from meats like bacon, ham, and lunch meat. In all of my previous books, I've consistently pointed out that pork—America's "other white meat"—should be avoided because pigs were called "unclean" in Leviticus and Deuteronomy. God created pigs as scavengers—animals that survive just fine on any farm slop or water swill tossed their way. Pigs have a simple stomach arrangement: whatever a pig eats goes down the hatch, straight into the stomach, and out the back door in four hours max. They'll even eat their own excrement, if hungry enough.

Even if you decide to keep eating commercial beef instead of the organic version, I absolutely urge you to stop eating pork. Read Leviticus 11 and Deuteronomy 14 to learn what God said about eating clean versus unclean animals, where Hebrew words used to describe "unclean meats" can be translated as "foul" and "putrid," the same terms the Bible uses to describe human waste.

The healthiest meat is fish caught in the wild, including salmon, sardines, herring, mackerel, tuna, snapper, bass, and cod. Wild-caught fish are a rich source of omega-3 fatty acids, which are also good for heart health. Researchers have found that when your body doesn't receive a sufficient supply of omega-3 fatty acids, the body uses saturated fat to construct cell membranes. These cell membranes, however, are less elastic, which has a negative effect on the heart because it's harder for the heart muscle to return to a resting rate.

One of the first associations between omega-3 fatty acids and human health happened in the 1970s when scientists studying the Inuit people of Greenland discovered that Inuits suffered far less coronary heart disease than Europeans, even though their diet was off-the-chart high in fat from eating whale, seal, and salmon.[9]

Please realize that not all sea life is healthy to eat. Shellfish and fish without fins and scales, such as catfish, shark, and eel, are also described in Leviticus 11 and Deuteronomy 14 as "unclean meats." God called hard-shelled crustaceans such as lobsters, crabs, shrimp, and clams unclean because they are "bottom feeders," content to sustain themselves on excrement from other fish. To be sure, this purifies water but does nothing for the health of their flesh—or yours, if you eat them.

Eating unclean foods fouls the body and may lead to increases in heart disease and cancer by introducing toxins into the blood-stream. God declared these meats unclean because He under-stands the ramifications of eating them, and you should as well.

2. Dairy products

Medical doctors lump the saturated fats in dairy products in the same category as red meat, implicating the fat intake as one of the key factors behind cardiovascular disease. Thus, doctors recommend that we should not eat full-fat dairy products. When reaching for a half gallon of milk at the supermarket, they say, be sure to choose a low-fat version like 2 percent or skim milk.

I don't see things the same way because I have never heard of a milking cow or goat producing 2 percent or skim milk. Reduced fat milk is less nutritious, less digestible, and can cause allergies. When it comes to preventing heart disease, I recom-mend that you purchase dairy products derived from goat's milk and sheep's milk rather than cow's milk, although dairy products from organic or grass-fed cows can be excellent as well. The reason I prefer goat's milk and goat's cheese lies in the goat milk's structure: its fat and protein molecules are tiny in size, which allows for rapid absorption in the digestive tract. Goat's milk is less allergenic because it does not contain the same complex proteins found in cow's milk. I also recommend you consume milk in its cultured or fermented form such as yogurt and kefir. The fermentation process makes the milk easier to digest, and its nutrients are more useable by the body.

Finally, let me address one more dairy product that directly relates to heart health but maybe not the way you think it does—eggs. When someone has a heart attack, one of the first items they're told to strike off their grocery list is eggs, because the high cholesterol levels are supposedly bad for their hearts.

That advice never made sense to me because eggs are a wonderful food deserving Hall of Fame status. This nutrient-dense food packs six grams of protein, a bit of vitamin B_{12}, vitamin E, lutein, riboflavin, folic acid, calcium, zinc, iron, and essential fatty acids into a mere seventy-five calories. The Harvard School of Public Health agrees with me.

Citing research by Harvard scientists, the Harvard School of Public Health says that moderate egg consumption—meaning one a day—does not increase heart risk in healthy individuals, and nutrients such as vitamins B_{12} and D, along with riboflavin and folate, help lower the risk of heart disease.[10] The Los Angeles Atherosclerosis Study found that the more eggs their subjects ate, the better their arteries looked.[11]

I believe you can safely eat two eggs a day, but I strongly urge you to buy high omega-3 eggs, which have become much more available in response to consumer demand. Natural food markets stock them, of course, but you'll also find omega-3 eggs at major supermarket chains as well as warehouse clubs like Costco.

Finally, I urge you not to overlook cultured dairy products, such as yogurt and kefir, which provide an excellent source of easily digestible protein, B vitamins, calcium, and probiotics.

3. Fruits and vegetables (and their juices)

This has to be the biggest no-brainer of all: everyone involved with cardiovascular disease, from the top medical specialists to those promoting alternative cures, sing from the same song sheet: You need to up your fruit and veggie consumption to prevent or battle heart disease. Yet the average American consumes far less than the recommended five to nine servings of fruits and vegetables daily, which is too bad. A Harvard School of Public Health study showed that for every extra serving of fruits and vegetables participants added to their diets, their risk of heart disease dropped by 4 percent.[12]

Fruits and veggies contain compounds that significantly lower blood pressure and cholesterol levels, which makes sense since fruits and vegetables are loaded with heart-healthy vitamins, minerals, fiber, and antioxidants. The pigments that color vegetables a dark green or orange are known as carotenoids, which are precursors to vitamin A and act as powerful antioxidants that can protect the body from cell damage caused by a specific type of oxygen molecules known as free radicals. The damage to cells caused by free radicals is thought to lead to heart disease.

You should eat a minimum of two or three fresh fruits daily, which can be consumed during snack time. For heart health, I recommend blueberries, cranberries, raspberries, and grapes, which contain flavonoids and reseveratrol, the latter being a phytoalexin that's been shown to be effective in the prevention of heart diseases.

A form of fermented grape juice—red wine—has been studied for decades in relation to cardiovascular disease. Does drinking a glass of red wine a day keep the cardiologist away? The American Heart Association reports that many studies have been published in scientific journals showing how drinking small amounts of red wine is good for the heart, leading newspaper editors to write cheery headlines ("'A Good Red Is Good for Your Heart,' Doctors Say").

Anyone who's vacationed in France, which I've been fortunate to do, has seen firsthand how any self-respecting Frenchman wearing a blue beret wouldn't think of sitting down in a restaurant without ordering a bottle of Bordeaux. The French have the highest per-capita consumption of wine in the world, eat a diet loaded with butter, cheese, cream, meats, and rich pâtés like *foie gras*, and many of them smoke cigarettes, yet they have a much lower rate of coronary heart disease than Americans. Even worse—or better, depending upon your perspective—is the news that deadly heart attacks claim half the victims in France as they do in the United States. No wonder this phenomenon is known as the "French Paradox."

Even though I don't drink alcohol as a rule (I sip half a glass a couple of times a year), I can see the healthy heart benefits that come from drinking a few ounces of red wine with dinner. Thus, I recommend organic wines that are preservative- and sulfite-free. Careful, though: if there was ever a double-edged sword, it would be alcohol. The overconsumption of booze has devastated relationships and wrecked millions of families over the years.

4. Soaked and sprouted seeds and grains

Like fruits and vegetables, whole grains, seeds, nuts, and breads made with sprouted or sour-leavened grains are heart-healthy foods. Apparently, the fiber, vitamins, phytochemicals, and antioxidants in properly prepared whole grains—wheat, spelt, kamut, quinoa, amaranth, millet, buckwheat, barley, corn, oats, and rice—appear to work together in the fight against deadly heart disease. "Whole grain" means the bran and germ are left on the grain during processing. "Soaked and sprouted grains" retain their plant enzymes when they are not cooked and are more digestible when cooked or baked.

5. Cultured and fermented vegetables

Often greeted with upturned noses at the dinner table, fermented vegetables such as sauerkraut, pickled carrots, beets, or cucumbers help reestablish the natural balance of our digestive system. Fermented vegetables like sauerkraut are brimming with vitamins, such as vitamin C, and contain almost four times the nutrients as unfermented cabbage.

The Japanese, who enjoy the second-longest life span in the

world and lower rates of heart disease than the U.S., eat fermented vegetables such as pickled cabbage, eggplant, and daikon radish with all their traditional meals.

6. Nuts

The Food and Drug Administration announced in 2003 that "scientific evidence suggests but does not prove that eating 1.5 ounces per day of most nuts, as part of a diet low in saturated fat and cholesterol, may reduce the risk of heart disease."[13]

I counted five qualifiers in that sentence, so the FDA wasn't treading too far out on a limb. But I've read plenty of research, including a Penn State study, showing that eating almonds, brazil nuts, cashews, hazelnuts, macadamia nuts, pecans, pistachios, walnuts, and lowly peanuts has a strong protective effect against coronary disease.[14] Nuts are a rich source of unsaturated fatty acids and plant-source omega-3—the "good" fat.

7. Spices

One of the first things cardiologists recommend for heart-attack victims is to clear away the table salt and other prepared seasonings that are major sources of sodium. What sodium does is make the body hold on to fluids, which causes the heart to work harder as it pumps the added fluids inside the body.

Not only do you not need salt to season your food, but your taste buds will learn to appreciate the vast array of healthy spices that you can employ while cooking and barbecuing. Two household spices in your cupboard may have heart-healthy properties. Ginger, the world's most widely cultivated spice, contains natural chemicals that discourage blood clotting, lower cholesterol, and increases the force or strength of heart muscle tissue. "Ginger offers a profound antioxidant principal action and observed effects, which include strengthening of the cardiac muscle and lowering of serum cholesterol," wrote Paul Schulick, author of *Ginger: Common Spice & Wonder Drug.* Schulick added that he knew of an Israeli hospital where coronary patients were counseled to take a one-half teaspoon daily of powdered ginger. That'll clear your nasal cavities![15]

There's another household spice that you should look for ways to use, but this one you won't be able to spoon into your mouth. I'm talking about cayenne pepper, which is rich in organic calcium and potassium, making it good for the heart. Cayenne pepper contains a high amount of beta-carotene, an antioxidant that lowers bad LDL cholesterol levels.

8. Water

Water isn't a food, of course, but this calorie-free and sugar-free substance performs many vital tasks for the body: regulating the body temperature, carrying nutrients and oxygen to the cells, cushioning joints, protecting organs and tissue, and removing toxins.

When it comes to heart health, drinking enough water ranks right at the top. "Basically, not drinking enough water can be as harmful to your heart as smoking," warned Jacqueline Chan, a doctor of public health and principle investigator behind a major Loma Linda University study that found that drinking high levels of water—five or more glasses a day—can significantly lower the risk of coronary heart disease.[16]

Water provides the viscosity in blood and plasma, almost like the lubricating effects of oil in a high-powered engine. Water helps move nutrients to our cells and helps keep cholesterol levels down. Not drinking enough water is bad for your body and your heart. F. Batmanghelidj, MD, author of *You're Not Sick, You're Thirsty!*, said that high cholesterol is a direct consequence of chronic dehydration. "In chronic dehydration, additional amounts of cholesterol will continue to be produced by the liver cells," he wrote.[17]

You should drink a minimum of eight glasses of water a day to stay hydrated. Sure, you'll go to the bathroom more often, but is that so bad? Drinking plenty of water is not only healthy for the body, but it's a key part of the Great Physician's Rx for a Healthy Heart Battle Plan (see page 71), so keep a water bottle close by and drink water before, during, and in between meals.

This seems a good place to talk about this country's obsession with coffee and tea, thanks to your neighborhood Starbucks. The American Heart Association says that the question of whether high caffeine intake increases the risk of coronary heart disease is still under study, but I must point out that coffee and tea have been consumed for thousands of years by some of the world's healthiest people. Although I'm not a coffee drinker myself, I will say that fresh-ground organic coffee flavored with organic cream and honey is fine when consumed in moderation, meaning one cup per day. Teas and herbal infusions (the latter beverage is made from herbs and spices, rather than the actual tea plant) are a better story altogether.

You'll find in my Great Physician's Rx for a Healthy Heart

Battle Plan (see page 71) that I recommend a cup of hot tea and honey with breakfast, dinner, and during snack time. I also advise consuming freshly made iced tea, as tea can be consumed hot or steeped and iced. Please note that while herbal tea provides many great health benefits, nothing can replace pure water for hydration. Although you can safely and healthfully consume two to four cups per day of tea and herbal infusions, you still need to drink at least six cups of pure water for all the good reasons I've described in this section.

WHAT NOT TO EAT

Whether you're trying to avoid a heart attack or you're recovering from one, here is a list of foods that should never find a way onto your plate or into your hands. I call them "The Deadly Dozen." Some I've already discussed elsewhere in this chapter, while the rest are presented here with a short commentary:

- **Processed meat and pork products.** These meats top my list because they are staples in the standard American diet and extremely unhealthy.

- **Shellfish and fish without fins and scales, such as catfish, shark, and eel.** Am I saying *au revoir* to lobster thermidor and *sayonara* to shrimp tempura? That's what I'm saying.

- **Hydrogenated oils.** This means margarine and shortening are taboo, as well as any commercial cakes, pastries, desserts, and anything with the words hydrogenated or partially hydrogenated on the label. Hydrogenated oils contain trans fatty acids, which can lead to arterial inflammation, one of the major risk factors for heart disease.

- **Artificial sweeteners.** Aspartame (found in NutraSweet and Equal), saccharin (Sweet'N Low), and sucralose (Splenda) are chemicals several hundred times sweeter than sugar. Do they cause cancer? Hard to say. At one time, diet drinks and sugar-free gum with saccharin once came with warning labels—"Use of this product may be hazardous to your health"—but the FDA took saccharin off the list of known carcinogens in 2000. In my book, however, artificial sweeteners should be completely avoided whether they come in blue, pink, or yellow packets.

- **White flour.** White flour isn't a problematic chemical like artificial sweeteners, but it's virtually worthless and not healthy for you.

- **White sugar.** If you're looking for a culprit to blame for bellies hanging over belt lines, then look no further.

- **Soft drinks.** Nothing more than liquefied sugar. A twenty-ounce bottle of Coke or Pepsi is the equivalent of eating fifteen teaspoons of sugar. Diet drinks loaded with artificial sweeteners are even worse.

- **Corn syrup.** Another version of sugar and just as bad for you, if not worse.

- **Pasteurized homogenized skimmed milk.** Like I said, whole organic, non-homogenized milk is better, and goat's milk is best.

- **Hydrolyzed soy protein.** Hydrolyzed soy protein is found in imitation meat products such as imitation crab. I would look at hydrolyzed soy protein like I would regard meat cured with nitrites: stay away from it. You're always going to be better off eating organic meats.

- **Artificial flavors and colors.** These are never good for you under the best of circumstances, and certainly not when you're battling to come back after a heart attack.

- **Anything fried in unhealthy oils.** Fried foods and heart-attack victims go together like . . . cheeseburgers topped with bacon.

EAT: WHAT FOODS ARE EXTRAORDINARY,
AVERAGE, OR TROUBLE?

I've prepared a comprehensive list of foods that are ranked in descending order based on their health-giving qualities. Foods at the top of the list are healthier than those at the bottom. The best foods to serve and eat are what I call "Extraordinary," which God created for us to eat and will give you the best chance to live a long and happy life. If you are battling cardiovascular disease, it's best if at least 75 percent of your diet is made up of foods from the Extraordinary category.

Foods in the Average category should make up less than 25

percent of your daily diet. If you're suffering or recovering from cardiovascular disease, these foods should be consumed sparingly.

Foods in the Trouble category should be consumed with extreme caution. If you're dealing with cardiovascular disease or on the mend after a heart attack, you should avoid these foods completely.

For the listing of Extraordinary, Average, and Trouble Foods, visit www.BiblicalHealthInstitute.com and click on "What to E.A.T."

℞ THE GREAT PHYSICIAN'S RX FOR A HEALTHY HEART: EAT TO LIVE

- *Eat only foods God created.*

- *Eat foods in a form that is healthy for the body.*

- *Consume foods high in omega-3 fatty acids.*

- *Consume foods high in fiber.*

- *Increase consumption of raw fruits and vegetables.*

- *Increase consumption of foods high in folic acid, vitamin B_{12}, and B_6, such as leafy greens, grass-fed red meat, and high omega-3 eggs.*

- *Practice fasting one day per week.*

- *Drink eight or more glasses of pure water per day.*

- *Avoid foods high in sugar.*

- *Avoid foods containing hydrogenated oils.*

Take Action

To learn how to incorporate the principles of eating to live into your daily life, please turn to page 71 for the Great Physician's Rx for a Healthy Heart Battle Plan.

KEY #2

Supplement Your Diet with Whole Food Nutritionals, Living Nutrients, and Superfoods

If you ask a doctor whether taking multivitamins and nutritional supplements are important in the prevention or treatment of heart disease, he or she will probably reply that a balanced diet is central, that no diet or nutritional plan can "cure" cardiovascular disease, and that taking vitamin or mineral supplements should never be considered a substitute for medical care. Your doctor will be backed up by the American Heart Association, which recommends eating a variety of foods in moderation, rather than taking supplements, although it makes an exception for omega-3 fatty acids.

This cautious recommendation is a form of defensive medicine that doesn't recognize the enormous potential of—and evidence for—nutritional supplements. Taking multivitamins and supplements can do more than cover your bases: they can keep you in the game against heart disease—and perhaps help you beat it.

One of the best heart-specific supplements you can take is called coenzyme Q10, which improves the supply of oxygen to the heart while supporting heart function and muscle strength. Coenzyme Q10 is found in every cell of the body and facilitates the activities of enzymes, but when you're put on a statin drug like Lipitor, coenzyme Q10 levels rapidly deplete. I recommend taking 50 milligrams of coenzyme Q10 three times a day to counteract the onerous side effects of these potent cholesterol-lowering drugs.

From the outset, though, please know that I'm not one who believes cardiovascular disease can be turned around with a bottle of pills. After years of study in naturopathic medicine and nutrition, I understand better than most that dietary supplements are just what they say they are—supplements, not a substitute for an inadequate diet and unhealthy lifestyle.

Still, nutritional supplements, living nutritionals, and superfoods are an important part of *The Great Physician's Rx for a Healthy Heart.* Topping my list are "whole food" or "living" multivitamins produced by adding vitamins and minerals to a living probiotic culture. These whole food vitamins and minerals contain different compounds such as organic acids, antioxidants, and key nutrients. They are more costly to produce since the ingredients—fruits, vegetables, sea vegetables, seeds, spices, vitamins and minerals, etc.—are put through a fermentation process similar to the digestive process of the body, but they are well worth the extra money.

If you're currently on heart medication, research suggests that you may be deficient in folic acid, vitamins B_{12} and B_6, and key minerals such as magnesium, vanadium, and chromium. As I mentioned in the last chapter, folic acid and vitamins B_{12} and B_6 play key roles in reducing high levels of homocysteine, which contribute to the artery-clogging process of atherosclerosis. Whole food nutritional supplements containing these important nutrients can address that situation as well as balance blood sugar levels, which improves metabolism.

In addition to a whole food or living multivitamin, you should also add the following supplements to your daily nutrition plan:

1. High omega-3 cod-liver oil

Remember how I talked about eating wild-caught fish because the meat is high in omega-3 fatty acids? Those with cardiovascular disease not only have high levels of fat in their blood, but they also travel through life with low levels of HDL, the "good" cholesterol. Sipping spoonfuls or taking liquid capsules of omega-3 cod-liver oil daily helps those with cardiovascular disease keep the high levels of fat in their blood cells—known as triglycerides—in check and may inhibit the progression of atherosclerosis.

If you can't stomach the thought of sipping omega-3 cod-liver oil, you can now take this important nutrient in easy-to-swallow liquid capsules (for recommended brands, visit www.Biblical HealthInstitute.com and click on the GPRx Resource Guide).

2. Green foods

The dislike of eating vegetables—especially green vegetables—follows many people into adulthood. They know that they *should* eat more vegetables, but they regard salads and vegetable servings as decorations to the main event—the meat and potatoes. Many people feel this way: the United States Department of Agriculture estimates that more than 90 percent of the U.S. population fails to eat the recommended three to five servings of vegetables each day.

I would hazard a guess that if you had a heart attack, then you're not a big vegetable eater—especially the green leafy kind. If you're having trouble motivating yourself to eat your veggies, I know a way your body can receive more green foods, which are important since they contain nutrients not found in the typical low-carb diet. I recommend the consumption of green super-food powders and caplets. All you do is mix the powder in water or your favorite juice or swallow a handful of caplets.

A good green food supplement is a certified organic blend of dried green vegetables, fermented vegetables, sea vegetables, microalgaes such as spirulina and chlorella, and sprouted grains and seeds. When you drink or swallow green foods, your body is taking in one of the most nutrient-dense foods on this green earth—but containing less than one-twentieth the calories of a Big Mac value meal. Superfoods are also an excellent source of folate, which protects you from developing heart disease.

3. Whole food fiber blend with flaxseeds

As mentioned in Key #1, fiber can be a heart patient's best friend since it lowers the bad LDL cholesterol levels. Consuming adequate fiber also improves regularity, which helps to efficiently eliminate toxins from the body. Since most of us receive about one-fifth of the optimal amount of fiber in our daily diet, I recommend taking a whole food fiber supplement. Look for one that supplies your body with a highly usable, vegetarian source of dietary fiber.

When searching for a fiber product that's right for you, choose a brand made from organic seeds, grains, and legumes that are fermented or sprouted for ease of digestion. (For recommended brands, visit www.BiblicalHealthInstitute.com and click on the GPRx Resource Guide.)

4. Probiotics

By definition, probiotics are living direct-fed microbials (DFMs) which promote the growth of beneficial or "friendly" bacteria in the intestinal tract. If you're experiencing constant intestinal pain, then supplement your diet with probiotics. The most effective probiotics contain soil-based organisms (SBOs), multiple strains of lactobacillus and bifidobacteria, and the friendly yeast saccharomyces boulardii. (For recommended brands, visit www.BiblicalHealthInstitute.com and click on the GPRx Research Guide.)

5. Enzymes

When you eat raw foods such as salad and fruit, you consume the enzymes they contain. When you eat cooked or processed meals, like from a restaurant kitchen, however, the body's pancreas must produce the enzymes necessary to digest them. The constant demand for enzymes strains the pancreas, which must kick in more enzymes to keep up with the demand. Without the proper levels of enzymes from foods—either raw or fermented—or from taking supplements, you are susceptible to heartburn, excessive gas and bloating, diarrhea, constipation, and low energy. Do these symptoms sound familiar?

If you're seeking to minimize the consumption of high-enzyme foods such as bananas, avocados, seeds, and grapes—which are high in sugars as well—then take plant-based digestive enzymes to ease the digestion of the food. (For recommended brands, visit www.BiblicalHealthInstitute.com and click on the GPRx Resource Guide.)

℞ THE GREAT PHYSICIAN'S RX FOR A HEALTHY HEART: SUPPLEMENT YOUR DIET

- *Take a whole food living multivitamin with each meal.*

- *Consume one to three teaspoons or three to nine capsules of omega-3 cod-liver oil per day.*

- *Take a whole food fiber / green food blend with beta-glucans from soluble oat fiber twice per day, morning and evening.*

- *Take an antioxidant / energy product with B vitamins, folic acid, and chromium with each meal.*

- *If you want improved digestion, take enzymes and probiotics.*

Take Action

To learn how to incorporate the principles of supplementing your diet with whole food nutritionals, living nutrients, and superfoods into your daily life, please turn to page 71 for the Great Physician's Rx for a Healthy Heart Battle Plan.

KEY #3

Practice Advanced Hygiene

I will be the first to admit that dipping your face into a basin of facial solution, cleaning under your fingernails with a special soap, or washing your hands after going to the bathroom doesn't sound like it has much to do with cardiovascular disease. But there's an aspect to good hygiene that's relevant to this discussion, and it has to do with the link between respiratory infections and various heart problems.

First, a little high school biology lesson.

Every day of your life, your body wards off gazillions of germs that break down your immune system and make you more susceptible to health problems. Every *other* day of your life (or so it seems), little "ow-ees" happen: a badly stubbed toe, mosquito bite, slight sunburn, pulled muscle, or nick while shaving your legs (for you gals) or your face (for you guys). Whenever any of these scenarios happen, the body mounts an instantaneous defense, sending cells and natural chemicals to assault those nasty flu germs or repair the slight gash in your skin. Scientifically speaking, this response is known as *inflammation.*

"Inflammation has become one of the hottest areas of medical research," wrote Christine Gorman and Alice Park in *Time* magazine. "Hardly a week goes by without the publication of yet another study uncovering a new way that chronic inflammation does harm to the body. It destabilizes cholesterol deposits in the coronary arteries, leading to heart attacks . . ."[1]

Most people think inflammation is something that happens to your back after spending an entire Saturday morning digging up weeds. Actually, inflammation occurs internally as well. When viruses invade the respiratory system by breathing in toxins from the air or by wolfing down a bad hot dog from the street vendor, the body launches a counterattack that lays waste to outside intruders and repairs any infected bodily organs.

When inflammation occurs, the liver produces a protein known as high-sensitivity C-reactive protein. This natural chemical is released into the bloodstream to help the body fight flu germs, for example, or repair itself after you pull a splinter out of your index finger. What medical researchers are learning, however, is that high C-reactive protein levels can be a warning sign of an impending heart attack. This is noteworthy because only 50 percent of the people who have heart attacks in the U.S. either have normal or moderately elevated cholesterol levels. High levels of C-reactive protein may also explain why people with low cholesterol develop heart disease in the first place. My third key, "Practice advanced hygiene," can protect your body from becoming chronically inflamed, which will lower your C-reactive protein levels as well as lower your risk of developing heart disease.

What do I mean by the phrase "advanced hygiene"?

I'm glad you asked, because I'm a great believer in protecting myself from harmful germs, and I've been practicing an advanced hygiene protocol for more than a decade. I've witnessed the results in my own life: no lingering head colds, no nagging sinus infections, no acute respiratory illnesses to speak of for many years, and a healthy heart.

I follow a program first developed by an Australian scientist, Kenneth Seaton, PhD, who discovered that ear, nose, throat, and skin problems could be linked to the fact that humans constantly touch their nose, eyes, and mouth with germ-carrying fingernails throughout the day.

In scientific terms, this is known as auto- or self-inoculation. So how do your fingernails get dirty? Through hand-to-hand contact with surfaces and other people. If you thought that most germs were spread by airborne exposure—someone sneezing at your table—you would be wrong. "Germs don't fly; they hitchhike," Dr. Seaton declared, and he's right.

Dr. Seaton estimates that once you pick up hitchhiking germs, they hibernate and hide around the fingernails, no matter how short you keep them trimmed.

A Primer on Washing Your Hands

1. Wet your hands with warm water. It doesn't have to be anywhere near scalding hot.

2. Apply plenty of soap into the palms of both hands. The best soap to use is a semisoft soap that you can dig your fingernails into.

3. Rub your hands vigorously together and scrub all the surfaces. Pay attention to the skin between the fingers and work the soap into the fingernails.

4. Rub and scrub for fifteen to thirty seconds, or about the time it takes to slowly sing "Happy Birthday to You."

5. Rinse well and dry your hands on a paper towel or clean cloth towel. If you're in a public restroom, it's a good idea to turn off the running water with the towel in your hand. An even *better* idea is to use that same towel to open the door since that door handle is the first place that non-washers touch after they've gone to the bathroom.

6. Keep waterless sanitizers in your purse or wallet in case soap and water are not available in the public restroom. These towelettes, although not ideal, are better than nothing.

How do you get germs on your hands? By shaking hands with others or touching things they touched: handrails, door-knobs, shopping carts, paper money, coins, and food. I know this stuff isn't pleasant dinnertime conversation, but practicing advanced hygiene has become an everyday habit for me. Since I'm aware that 90 percent of germs take up residence around my fingernails, I use a creamy semisoft soap rich in essential oils. Each morning and evening, I dip both of my hands into the tub of semisoft soap and dig my fingernails into the cream. Then I work the special cream around the tips of my fingers, cuticles, and fingernails for fifteen to thirty seconds. When I'm finished, I rinse my hands under running water, lathering them for fifteen seconds before rinsing. After my hands are clean, I take another dab of semisoft soap and wash my face.

When to Wash Your Hands

- After you go to the bathroom
- Before and after you insert and remove contact lenses
- Before and after food preparation
- Before you eat
- After you sneeze, cough, or blow your nose
- After cleaning up after your pet
- After handling money
- After changing a diaper
- After blowing a child's nose
- After handling garbage
- After cleaning your toilets
- After shaking a bunch of hands
- After shopping at the supermarket
- After attending an event at a public theater
- Before and after sexual intercourse

My second step involves a procedure that I call a "facial dip." I fill my washbasin or a clean large bowl with warm but not hot water. When enough water is in the basin, I add one to two tablespoons of regular table salt and two eyedroppers of a mineral-based facial solution into the cloudy water. I mix everything up with my hands, and then I bend over and dip my face into the cleansing matter, opening my eyes several times to allow the membranes to be cleansed. After coming up for air, I dunk my head a second time and blow bubbles through my nose. I call it "sink snorkeling."

My final two steps of advanced hygiene involve the application of very dilute drops of hydrogen peroxide and minerals into my ears for thirty to sixty seconds to cleanse the ear canal, followed by brushing my teeth with an essential oil tooth solution to cleanse my teeth, gums, and mouth of unhealthy germs. (For a listing of my favorite advanced hygiene products, visit www.BiblicalHealth Institute.com and click on the GPRx Resource Guide.)

Speaking of dental hygiene, medical research has found that people with periodontal (or gum) disease are almost twice as likely to suffer from coronary heart disease.[2] One theory is that oral bacteria enters the bloodstream and affects the heart by attaching to fatty plaques in the coronary arteries.

Brushing your teeth well and regularly practicing advanced hygiene involves discipline; you have to remind yourself to do it until it becomes an ingrained habit. I find it easier to follow these steps in the morning when I'm freshly awake than later in the evening when I'm tired and bleary-eyed—although I do my best to practice advanced hygiene morning and evening and hardly ever miss. Either way, I know it only takes three minutes or so to complete all of the advanced hygiene steps, and those might be the best three minutes a day for your heart.

Finally, there's another protein floating around in your bloodstream that you should know about, and it happens to be the most abundant one. It's called albumin, and this protein transports hormones, nutrients, and wastes in your bloodstream. Like dump trucks on their way to the landfill, albumin hauls waste and toxic cells to the liver for degradation and elimination from the body.

Medical researchers have also discovered another interesting bit of news: high albumin levels may be critically important to the prevention of diseases like cardiovascular disease. Heart-attack patients, when tested, have low albumin levels, according to Dr. Seaton. How this relates to heart disease is still being researched, but doctors believe that those with low albumin levels at the time a heart attack strikes could be at greater risk.

Dr. Seaton is certain that albumin levels are linked to *hygiene*, not diet, meaning that albumin levels can be optimized by practicing advanced hygiene, which underscores the importance of this key as part of *The Great Physician's Rx for a Healthy Heart*.

R₂ THE GREAT PHYSICIAN'S RX FOR A HEALTHY HEART: PRACTICE ADVANCED HYGIENE

- *Dig your fingers into a semisoft soap with essential oils and wash your hands regularly, paying special attention to removing germs from underneath your fingernails.*

- *Cleanse your nasal passageways and the mucous membranes of the eyes daily by performing a facial dip.*

- *Cleanse the ear canals at least twice per week.*

- *Use an essential oil-based tooth solution daily to remove germs from the teeth, gums, and mouth.*

Take Action

To learn how to incorporate the principles of practicing advanced hygiene into your daily life, please turn to page 71 for the Great Physician's Rx for a Healthy Heart Battle Plan.

Key #4

Condition Your Body
with Exercise and Body Therapies

When I reached toddlerhood, I darted around the house like the Roadrunner, zooming from one room to the next until my pooped parents tucked me in bed. I turned two years old in 1977, the year the "jogging craze" was sweeping the country. Outside my home, the sidewalks were packed with baby boomers in their twenties and thirties running in floppy T-shirts, fluorescent-colored shorts, and first-generation Nikes. (Dad and Mom weren't pounding the pavement, though. Jogging wasn't their thing.)

The pied piper leading the pack was Jim Fixx, author of *The Complete Book of Running*. Upon its publication in 1977, Fixx's book, which trumpeted the health benefits of running, became the best-selling nonfiction hardcover book ever. Fixx was credited with launching the running boom.

Seven years later, Jim Fixx collapsed and died of a heart attack while running along a tree-shaded road in Vermont. Talk about life's ironies; he was only fifty-two years old. Although he's been gone for more than two decades, Fixx's name still pops up in crossword puzzles (Clue: Dead runner. Four letters).

Jim Fixx's sad story is also a cautionary tale: when it comes to heart health, vigorous exercise may prove too stressful for hearts with undiscovered coronary disease, but if you lead a sedentary life, you're doomed as well. The heart is your ultimate muscle, and exercise preserves and protects the quality of the heart's blood vessels and prevents heart attacks. Regular, consistent exercise almost always does a heart good. You'll live longer, lower blood pressure, and improve blood circulation.

When it comes to cardiovascular disease and Key #4, "Condition Your Body with Exercise and Body Therapies," you don't want to wait for chest pains, elevated cholesterol levels, or surviving a first heart attack to get your attention. There might not be a next time. And if you're a heart-attack survivor, there's a pool of studies showing that people who begin regular physical activity after a coronary blockage have better survival rates and quality of life.

I have a background in physical fitness, having been a certified fitness trainer. If you were my client, having been informed by your doctor that you must begin an exercise program, I would start you with *functional fitness*. This form of gentle exercise raises your heartbeat, strengthens the body's core muscles, and exercises the cardiovascular system through the performance of real-life activities in real-life positions.

Functional fitness can be done with no equipment or by employing dumbbells, mini-trampolines, and stability balls. You can find functional fitness classes and equipment at gyms around the country, including LA Fitness, Bally Total Fitness, and local YMCAs. You'll be asked to perform squats with feet apart, feet together, and one back with the other forward. You'll be asked to do reaching lunges, push-ups against a wall, and "supermans" that involve lying on the floor and lifting up your right arm while lifting your left leg into a fully extended position. What you *won't* be asked to perform are high-impact exercises like those found in pulsating aerobics classes. (For more information on functional fitness, visit www.GreatPhysiciansRx.com.)

I would also incorporate these forms of exercise and body therapies:

Take up weight training. This is a form of anaerobic exercise that strengthens and develops muscle tissue. Pushing plates at your local health club twice a week for thirty minutes at a time is a good start for your heart, but three times a week would be superior if you're making a lifestyle change. Leave the power lifting to the young bucks, however.

Become a "rebounder." Rebounders look like mini-trampolines, are great for low-impact exercise, and burn more calories than jogging. One of rebounding's special benefits is its ability to improve flow in the lymphatic system.

Practice deep-breathing exercises. Most of the time, we don't completely fill the diaphragm with air because we're not aware that our lungs hang all the way toward the bottom of the rib cage. I recommend sitting in a chair and concentrating on filling the lungs completely. Count to five as you breathe in, and then hold your breath for several seconds before exhaling through your mouth for several more seconds. Visualize the diaphragm moving up and down as your lungs expand. Deep-breathing techniques are peaceful, powerful tools to calm your nervous system, slow down your heartbeat, and restore your energy.

Walk up a storm. Walking is especially good for those who've been lax in working out over the years. This low-impact route to fitness places a gentle strain on the hips and the rest of the body, and when done briskly, makes the heart work harder and expend more energy.

Best of all, you can walk when it fits your schedule—before work, on your lunch hour, before dinner, after dinner, etc. You set the pace; you decide how much you put into this exercise. Walking is a great social exercise that allows you to carry on a civilized conversation with a friend or loved one.

Go to bed earlier. Sleep is a body therapy in short supply these days. A nationwide "sleep deficit" means that we're packing in as much as we can from the moment we wake up until we crawl into bed sixteen, seventeen, or eighteen exhausting hours later. American adults are down to a little less than seven hours of sleep each night, a good two hours less than our great-great-grandparents slept a hundred years ago. This can't be good for the heart.

How many hours of sleep are you getting nightly? The sleep experts say the magic number is eight. That's because when people are allowed to sleep as much as they would like in a con-trolled setting, like in a sleep laboratory, they naturally sleep eight hours in a twenty-four-hour time period.

This is a good time to talk about sleep apnea and how it relates to heart health. Sleep apnea is a serious, potentially life-threatening condition characterized by brief interruptions in breathing during sleep. Those with sleep apnea are often unaware that they wheeze and snore throughout the night, only to have their breathing suddenly stop for a long moment. You can only imagine the havoc that low oxygen levels wreck on the heart and lungs—or worry your spouse. If your snoring knocks family photos off the wall, or your spouse comments about momentary pauses in your breathing, seek medical attention right away. You may require a special pressure-generating machine to survive the night.

Rest on the seventh day. In addition to proper sleep, the body needs a time of rest every seven days to recharge its batteries. This is accomplished by taking a break from the rat race on Saturday or Sunday. God created the earth and the heavens in six days and rested on the seventh, giving us an example and a reminder that we need to take a break from our labors. Otherwise, we're prime candidates for burnout.

Let the sun shine in. You may not see much correlation between sunning yourself and heart health, but let me explain. When your face or your arms and legs are exposed to sunlight, your skin synthesizes vitamin D from the ultraviolet rays of sunlight. The body needs vitamin D, which is not a vitamin but actually a critical hormone that helps regulate the health of more than thirty different tissues and organs, including the heart. I recommend intentionally exposing yourself to at least fifteen minutes of sunlight a day to increase vitamin D levels in the body.

Treat yourself to hydrotherapy. Hydrotherapy comes in the form of baths, showers, washing, and wraps—using hot *and* cold water. For instance, I wake up with a hot shower in the mornings, but then I turn off the hot water and stand under the brisk cold water for about a minute, which totally invigorates me. Cold water stimulates the body and boosts oxygen use in the cells, while hot water dilates blood vessels, which improves blood circulation and transports more oxygen to the brain.

Sitting in a sauna or taking a steam bath are other forms of hydrotherapy that boost cardiovascular circulation. I highly recommend that you find a way to add these body therapies to your weekly schedule.

Finally, pamper yourself with aromatherapy and music therapy. In aromatherapy, essential oils from plants, flowers, and spices are introduced to your skin and pores either by rubbing them in or inhaling their aromas. The use of these essential oils will not miraculously repair blocked coronary arteries, but they will give you an emotional lift. Try rubbing a few drops of myrtle, coriander, hyssop, galbanum, or frankincense onto your palms, and then cup your hands over your mouth and nose and inhale. A deep breath will invigorate the spirit.

So will listening to soft and soothing music that promotes relaxation and healing. I know what I like when it comes to music therapy: contemporary praise and worship music. No matter what works for you, you'll find that listening to uplifting "mood" music can heal the body, soul, and spirit.

THE GREAT PHYSICIAN'S RX FOR A HEALTHY HEART: CONDITION YOUR BODY WITH EXERCISE AND BODY THERAPIES

℞

- Make a commitment and an appointment to exercise for at least one hour three times a week or more.

- Incorporate five to fifteen minutes of functional fitness into your daily schedule.

- Take a brisk walk and see how much better you feel at the end of the day.

- Make a conscious effort to practice deep-breathing exercises once a day. Inflate your lungs to full and hold for several seconds before slowly exhaling.

- Go to bed earlier, paying close attention to how much sleep you get before midnight. Do your best to get eight hours of sleep nightly. Remember that sleep is the most important nonnutrient you can incorporate into your health regimen.

- End your next shower by changing the water temperature to cool (or cold) and standing underneath the spray for one minute.

- Next Saturday or Sunday, take a day of rest. Dedicate the day to the Lord and do something fun and relaxing that you haven't done in a while. Make your rest day work free, errand free, and shopping free. Trust God that He'll do more with His six days than you can do with seven.

- During your next break from work, sit outside in a chair and face the sun. Soak up the rays for ten or fifteen minutes.

- Incorporate essential oils into your daily life.

- Play worship music in your home, in your car, or on your iPod. Focus on God's plan for your life.

Take Action

To learn how to incorporate the principles of conditioning your body with exercise and body therapies into your daily life, please turn to page 71 for the Great Physician's Rx for a Healthy Heart Battle Plan.

KEY #5

Reduce Toxins in Your Environment

D r. Dobson, who turned seventy years young in the spring of 2006, has a good thing going for him and his heart: he lives at altitude. Colorado Springs, Colorado, where he moved a year after his 1990 heart attack, is nestled against the Rocky Mountain's Front Range at 6,035 feet above sea level. Living at altitude gives the heart a good workout and enables the cardiovascular system to cope with lower levels of oxygen. This leaves me a bit envious since I live in a state where the highest "mountain," Britton Hill, is 345 feet high, and the tallest peak near my home is the Harriet Himmel Gilman Theater at West Palm Beach's CityPlace.

Dr. Dobson has another environmental factor in his heart's favor: he no longer lives in smoggy Southern California, where a thick blanket of air pollution often hovers over the L.A. basin. Air pollution is definitely a cause of heart disease, according to a study performed by the American Heart Association regarding the long-term effects of chronic exposure to pollution. In another study, researchers in Athens, Greece, collected daily values of primary air pollutants—smoke, sulfur dioxide, and auto emissions—from eight stations as well as data regarding the number of deaths due to heart disease. They were able to extrapolate a significant association between cardiovascular death and several air pollutants, so that's something to think about if you have serious heart problems.[1]

Moving to the Rocky Mountains, for example, isn't a cure-all since *indoor* air pollution can be hazardous to your heart, as well. The American Lung Association estimates that we spend 90 percent of our time indoors, breathing recirculated air-conditioned air in the summer and heated air in the winter—air swirling with toxic particles. Today's well-insulated homes and energy-efficient doors and windows trap "used" air filled with carbon dioxide, nitrogen dioxide, and pet dander. These pollutants trigger and accelerate narrowing of carotid arteries.

I recommend opening your doors and windows periodically to freshen the air you breathe, even if the temperatures are blazing hot or downright freezing. Just a few minutes of fresh air will do wonders. I also recommend the purchase of a quality air filter, which will remove and neutralize tiny airborne particles of dust, soot, pollen, mold, and dander. I have set up four high-quality air purifiers in our home that scrub harmful impurities out of the air.

Chemicals and toxins dangerous to heart health are also present in our food supply. If your blood and urine were tested, lab technicians would uncover dozens of toxins in your bloodstream, including PCBs (polychlorinated biphenyls), dioxins, furans, trace metals, phthalates, VOCs (volatile organic compounds), and chlorine.

Some toxins are water-soluble, meaning they are rapidly passed out of the body and present no harm. Unfortunately, many more toxins are fat soluble, meaning that it can take months or years before they are completely eliminated from your system. Some of the more well-known fat-soluble toxins are dioxins, phthalates, and chlorine, and when they are not eliminated from the body, they become stored in your fatty tissues and clog your arteries.

The best way to flush fat-soluble toxins out of your bloodstream is by increasing your intake of drinking water, which helps eliminate toxins through the kidneys. You must increase the fiber in your diet to eliminate toxins through the bowel, exercise and sweat to eliminate toxins through the lymphatic system, and practice deep breathing to eliminate toxins through the lungs.

Another way to reduce the number of toxins is to consume organic or grass-fed meat and dairy products. Remember, most commercially produced beef, chicken, and pork act as chemical magnets for toxins in the environment, so they will not be as healthy as grass-fed beef. In addition, consuming organic produce purchased at health food stores, roadside stands, and farmer's markets (only if produce is grown locally and unsprayed) will expose you to less pesticide residues, as compared to conventionally grown fruits and vegetables.

Typical canned tuna (also available in a soft pack) is another food to eat minimally, although many popular diets include tuna and salad as a lunchtime or dinner staple. Metallic particles of mercury, lead, and aluminum continue to be found in the fatty tissues of tuna, swordfish, and king mackerel. However, there is now a canned tuna available that is not only low in mercury but high in omega-3 fatty acids. This tuna can be safely consumed many times per week and contains the same amount of heart-healthy omega-3 fats (such as EPA and DHA) as fatty fish such as salmon and sardines. (For more information on low-mercury, high omega-3 tuna, visit www.BiblicalHealthInstitute.com and click on the GPRx Resource Guide.)

What to Drink

I've already touted the healthy benefits of drinking water, but when it comes to reducing toxins in your environment, water is especially important because of its ability to flush out toxins and other metabolic wastes from the body. Those with cardiovascular disease tend to have larger metabolic loads.

The importance of drinking enough water cannot be overstated: water is a life force involved in nearly every bodily process, from digestion to blood circulation. Your heart pumps blood much more efficiently when you're well hydrated.

The answer to hydration is not switching to diet soft drinks or beverages such as coffee, tea, and fruit juice, even though the latter can be healthy for you. Diet drinks contain artificial sweeteners like aspartame, acesulfame-K, or sucralose. Even though the Food and Drug Administration has approved the use of artificial sweeteners in drinks (and food), these chemical food additives may prove to be detrimental to your health in the long-term.

Nothing beats plain old water—a liquid created by God to be totally compatible with your body. You should be drinking the proverbial eight glasses of water daily.

I know what you're thinking: *Jordan, if I drink that much water, I can never be further than fifteen steps from a bathroom.*

Yes, you will probably triple your trips to the toilet, but trust me on this: if you're serious about having a healthy heart, you must be serious about drinking enough water. There's no other physiological way for you to rid yourself of fat reserves and toxins stored inside your body.

I don't recommend drinking water straight from the tap, however. Nearly all municipal water is routinely treated with chlorine or chloramine, potent bacteria-killing chemicals. I've installed a whole-house filtration system that removes the chlorine and other impurities out of the water *before* it enters our household pipes. My wife, Nicki, and I can confidently turn on the tap and enjoy the health benefits of chlorine-free water for drinking, cooking, and bathing. And since our water doesn't have a chemical aftertaste, we're more apt to drink it than we would be without the filtration system. (A less expensive approach would be to purchase a countertop water pitcher with a built in carbon-based filter for less than twenty dollars.)

Toxins Elsewhere in Your Environment

There are other toxins not directly related to cardiovascular disease but are important enough to mention:

- **Plastics.** Although I drink bottled water from plastic containers when I'm not at home, I think it's safer to drink water from glass cups because of the presence of dioxins and phthalates added in the manufacturing process of plastic.

- **Household cleaners.** Many of today's commercial house cleaners contain potentially harmful chemicals and solvents that expose people to VOCs—volatile organic compounds—which can cause eye, nose, and throat irritation. Nicki and I have found that natural ingredients like vinegar, lemon juice, and baking soda are excellent substances that make our home spic-and-span. Natural cleaning products that aren't harsh, abrasive, or potentially dangerous to your family are available in grocery and natural food stores.

- **Skin care and body-care products.** Toxic chemicals such as chemical solvents and phthalates are found in lipstick, lip gloss, lip conditioner, hair coloring, hair spray, shampoo, and soap. Ladies, when you rub a tube of lipstick across your lips, your skin readily absorbs these toxins, and that's unhealthy. As with the case regarding household cleaners, you can find natural cosmetics in progressive natural food markets, although they are becoming more widely available in drugstores and beauty stores.

- **Toothpaste.** A tube of toothpaste contains a warning that in case of accidental swallowing, you should contact the local Poison Control Center. What's that all about? Most commercially available toothpastes contain artificial sweeteners, potassium nitrate, sodium fluoride, and a whole bunch of long, unpronounceable words. Again, search out a healthy, natural version.

Finally, let me pull the guys aside for a moment and talk about heart health and . . . your sex life. If you've been having trouble . . . you know . . . performing, be aware that the American Heart Association reports a strong link between coronary artery disease and erectile dysfunction.

It's all in the blood pressure and the blood flow, so if you were looking for something else to inspire you other than staying alive, then let this be it.

R℟ THE GREAT PHYSICIAN'S RX FOR A HEALTHY HEART: REDUCE TOXINS IN YOUR ENVIRONMENT

- *Pay attention to the amount of air pollution—inside and outside your home—especially if you are fighting cardiovascular disease.*

- *Drink the recommended eight glasses of water daily—or one quart for every fifty pounds of body weight.*

- *Use glass containers instead of plastic containers whenever possible.*

- *Improve indoor air quality by opening windows and buying an air-filtration system.*

- *Use natural cleaning products for your home.*

• *Use natural products for skin care, body care, hair care, cosmetics, and toothpaste.*

Take Action

To learn how to incorporate the principles of reducing toxins in your environment, please turn to page 71 for the Great Physician's Rx for a Healthy Heart Battle Plan.

KEY #6

Avoid Deadly Emotions

That really touched my heart."

We've all heard—or mumbled—that phrase at one time or another, but have you ever thought about why people refer to the heart when they speak about their emotions? Or, put another way, why do we think emotions are centered in the heart?

"The emotions are centered in the brain, of course," wrote author Joel Achenbach. "But when we experience a powerful emotion—fear, anger, grief, love—adrenaline pours into the blood, which increases blood pressure and accelerates the heart. So it makes perfect sense to think the heart controls emotion. Otherwise, when we say the Pledge of Allegiance, we'd have to put our hand on our foreheads."[1] Wouldn't want to do that.

Throughout history, the heart has been called upon by psalmists, bards, and songwriters to describe emotions that are almost indescribable. "The LORD is my strength and my shield; my *heart* trusts in him, and I am helped. My *heart* leaps for joy and I will give thanks to him in song," wrote David in Psalm 28:7 (NIV, emphasis added).

A couple of thousand years later, Shakespeare penned, "Expectation is the root of all heartbreak"; and we can't forget that one of Elton John's monster hits is "Don't Go Breaking My Heart."

Singing about puppy love and broken hearts is a staple of pop music, but it's also a reminder that the connection between emotions and the state of the heart is real. My friend, Don Colbert, MD, author of the excellent book *Deadly Emotions*, says that researchers have directly and scientifically linked deadly emotions to cardiovascular disease and hypertension, and emotions such as anxiety and fear have been linked to heart palpitations.

Anger, acrimony, apprehension, agitation, anxiety, and alarm *are* deadly emotions, and when you experience any of these feelings—whether justified or not—they alter the chemistry in and around your heart muscle. Here's the picture that Dr. Colbert described:

> What happens in times of stress? Adrenaline is released into the bloodstream, causing the heart to speed up and beat harder. Adrenaline is also triggering the coronary arteries and the heart to dilate in an effort to deliver more oxygen and nutrients to the heart muscle. If the coronary arteries are filled with plaque, or if the coronary arterial walls have been thickened owing to high blood-pressure damage, then instead of dilating, the coronary arteries constrict.
>
> The heart then must beat even harder and faster. The end result is angina, a heart attack, arrhythmia, or the release of a blood clot that results in total blockage of a key vessel and sudden death.[2]

If feelings of anger or hostility are welling up inside, it's probably because someone has said something mean-spirited or has belittled you. Trust me: I know that words can hurt, and words can break a heart.

This is not the time to fall off the healthy food wagon or revert to eating fat-filled and high-sugar "comfort foods" sure to compound the problems in your cardiovascular system. This is the time to forgive those who've made your life miserable, made cutting remarks about you or your children, or done something to hurt your family financially.

If you've been hurt in the past by mean-spirited comments and people, I'm sure I'm not the first to urge you to put the past in the rearview mirror and move forward. But you must. If you follow the Great Physician's Rx for a healthy lifestyle, I'm confident that this will help you deal with any deadly emotions weighing on your mind. Please remember that no matter how bad you've been hurt in the past, it's still possible to forgive. "For if you forgive men their trespasses, your heavenly Father will also forgive you," Jesus said in Matthew 6. "But if you do not forgive men their trespasses, neither will your Father forgive your trespasses" (Matthew 6:14–15).

Give those who tormented you your forgiveness, and then let it go. Then memorize this wise advice from King Solomon: "A merry heart doeth good like a medicine" (Proverbs 17:22 KJV).

R℞ THE GREAT PHYSICIAN'S RX FOR A HEALTHY HEART: AVOID DEADLY EMOTIONS

- *Realize the damage to your heart when you're sad, scared, or stressed by everyday life.*

• *Trust God when you face circumstances that cause you to worry or become anxious.*

• *Practice forgiveness every day and forgive those who hurt you.*

Take Action

To learn how to incorporate the principles of avoiding deadly emotions into your daily life, please turn to page 71 for the Great Physician's Rx for a Healthy Heart Battle Plan.

KEY #7

Live a Life of Prayer and Purpose

A few years ago, I got into collecting baseball memorabilia. I purchased some Barry Bonds stuff, including a painting, a bat, and a ball signed by him. (The jury's out on what the Barry Bonds market will be like in coming years.) I also bought a large painting of "A-Rod"—New York Yankee third baseman Alex Rodriguez—which now occupies a sizeable wall in my office.

There's another Yankee great I enjoy, and his name is Yogi Berra, who squatted behind home plate for the Yankees from 1947 to 1963. Back in his playing days, Yogi was known as a thoughtful, intelligent catcher, despite the limitations of an eighth-grade education.

What makes Yogi special—and famous these days—is his uncanny ability to say something funny or farcical without batting an eye. If you asked Yogi what time it was, he'd reply, "You mean right now?" When someone asked him about a popular restaurant named Charlie's, Yogi deadpanned, "No one goes there anymore—it's too crowded."

On another occasion, Yogi's wife, Carmen, asked him a serious question. "Yogi, you are from St. Louis, we live in New Jersey, and you played ball in New York. If you go before I do, where would you like me to have you buried?"

"Surprise me," Yogi replied.

Finally, when referring to playing left field in Yankee Stadium, which was beset by early evening shadows, he quipped, "It gets late early out there."

I'm afraid that it gets late early for a lot of heart-attack victims, many who were blissfully traveling through life only to have their worlds turn suddenly black as they plunged into eternity. For those of us left behind, the pain of losing loved ones to sudden, near-instantaneous death is shocking and difficult to handle. This emotional issue certainly resonates with me, because both of my grandfathers succumbed to heart attacks when they were in their mid-fifties and early sixties.

When I was just seventeen months old, I lost my first grandfather, Papa Al, after his third heart attack in less than two years. My mother's father was first stricken while vacationing in Israel with my Grandma Rose. While strolling with a tour group toward the Temple Mount, chest pains seized him. An aneurism blew out one of his ventricles, but somehow he survived. He remained hospitalized in Israel for months before doctors cleared him to return to the U.S.

Papa Al was a prime candidate for a coronary bypass operation, but the operation wasn't nearly as routine then as it is these days. Cardiologists ruled him out as a candidate. Several months after returning from the Holy Land, my grandfather suffered a second myocardial infarction—another major heart attack. He survived this one as well, but barely. He remained couch-bound on oxygen until a third heart attack delivered the final deathblow.

Papa Al was only fifty-five years old.

As for my father's father, Joshua Rubin "Americanized" his name to Jerry to escape persecution for being a Jew. Grandpa Jerry had no problem adopting the all-American diet heavy in junk foods either. Before he went to bed, he liked to help himself to a huge helping of ice cream while dipping his right hand into a bag of salty pretzels. He bought Fudgsicles by the dozen and treated himself to Howard Johnson's every Friday night, where he purchased a sundae with egg cream. He frequented burger joints and always ordered big, creamy shakes and French fries.

Grandpa Jerry was an overweight dentist who never saw the doctor. He tipped the scales at well over 250 pounds on a six-foot-one apple-shaped frame. Although he never exercised, he was as strong as an ox and never sick.

When Grandpa Jerry retired from his successful dental practice at the age of sixty-one, he was ready to enjoy the golden years. He and Grandmother Anne purchased a retirement home in South Miami Beach. When I was nine years old, my parents received the type of ominous phone call that only seems to come at 2:00 in the morning: Grandpa Jerry had died of a sudden and massive coronary. He had been reading in bed when he fell asleep, only to wake up coughing and gasping for air. The end came quickly, and paramedics who arrived on the scene couldn't save him. The doctor who performed the autopsy said that he had rarely seen that much plaque in someone's arteries.

I wish I had had my grandfathers longer on this earth so that I could have gotten to know them better, but sharing their stories gives me a renewed sense of purpose to help people suffering from cardiovascular disease.

Heart disease is a horrible affliction that causes you to confront your mortality, and prayer is the most powerful tool we possess in the fight to keep a healthy heart. Prayer acknowledges that there is something . . . Someone . . . beyond the mortal confines of our lives. Talking to our Maker through prayer shouldn't be the treatment of last resort but of *first* resort. God may not answer our prayers in the way we expect Him to, but prayer will transform our hearts into greater alignment with His.

"Prayer must be foundational to every Christian endeavor," wrote Germaine Copeland, author of *Prayers That Avail Much*. Her book contains more than 150 prayers covering just about every situation under the sun: praying for relatives to receive Jesus as Lord and Savior, healing for damaged emotions, victory over depression, and victory over fear. I was particularly drawn to Mrs. Copeland's prayer for "letting go of the past":

Lord, I unfold my past and put into proper perspective those things that are behind. I trust in You, Lord, with all of my heart and lean not on my own understanding. Regardless of my past, I look forward to what lies ahead. I strain to reach the end of the race and receive the prize for which You are calling me up to heaven because of what Christ Jesus did for me. In His name I pray, amen.[1]

If you feel drawn to God at a crucial time like this, I urge you to get on your knees today. Prayer is imperative! Do not underestimate the power of communicating with your heavenly Father. When you pray and open up to God, you allow Him to fill your heart with Scripture, where He can speak to you in the stillness of the moment and transform your health simultaneously.

The possibility that sick people who are prayed for experience better recoveries has been the subject of studies in recent years. The first major study, in 1988, involved victims of heart attack, heart failure, and other cardiac problems at San Francisco General Hospital. Cardiologist Randolph Byrd, MD, assigned 192 patients in cardiac ICU to be prayed for by born-again Christians and 201 patients in cardiac ICU to be in the "not prayed for by anybody" cluster. Patients, doctors, and nurses did not know which group was which. The Christians who prayed were scattered around the country and given only first names, the diagnoses, and the prognoses of the patients. Dr. Byrd dramatically concluded that study found that patients who were prayed for needed far less medication and experienced fewer complications.[2]

Our Creator hears our prayers, which reminds me of something else that Yogi Berra is famous for saying:

"It ain't over till it's over."

℞ THE GREAT PHYSICIAN'S RX FOR A HEALTHY HEART: LIVE A LIFE OF PRAYER AND PURPOSE

- *Pray continually.*

- *Remember God's promises upon waking and before you retire.*

- *No matter where you are on your health journey, find God's purpose for your life and live it.*

Take Action

To learn how to incorporate the principles of living a life of prayer and purpose into your daily life, please turn to page 71 for the Great Physician's Rx for a Healthy Heart Battle Plan.

THE GREAT PHYSICIAN'S RX FOR A HEALTHY HEART BATTLE PLAN

Upon Waking

Prayer: thank God because this is the day that the Lord has made. Rejoice and be glad in it. Thank Him for the breath in your lungs and the life in your body. Ask the Lord to heal your body and use your experience to benefit the lives of others. Read Matthew 6:9–13 out loud.

Purpose: ask the Lord to give you an opportunity to add significance to someone's life today. Watch for that opportunity. Ask God to use you this day for His intended purpose.

Advanced hygiene: for hands and nails, jab fingers into semisoft soap four or five times, and lather hands with soap for fifteen seconds, rubbing soap over cuticles and rinsing under water as warm as you can stand. Take another swab of semisoft soap into your hands and wash your face. Next, fill basin or sink with water as warm as you can stand, and add one-to-three tablespoons of table salt and one to three eyedroppers of iodine-based mineral solution. Dunk face into water and open eyes, blinking repeatedly underwater. Keep eyes open underwater for three seconds. After cleaning your eyes, put your face back in the water, and close your mouth while blowing bubbles out of your nose. Come up from the water, and then immerse your face once again, gently taking water into your nostrils and expelling bubbles. Come up from the water, and blow your nose into facial tissue. To cleanse the ears, use hydrogen peroxide and mineral-based ear drops, putting two or three drops into each ear and letting stand for sixty seconds. Tilt your head to expel the drops. For the teeth, apply two or three drops of essential oil-based tooth drops to the toothbrush. This can be used to brush your teeth or added to existing toothpaste. After brushing your teeth, brush your tongue for fifteen seconds. (For recommended advanced hygiene products, visit www.BiblicalHealthInstitute.com and click on the GPRx Resource Guide.)

Reduce toxins: open your windows for one hour today. Use natural soap and natural skin and body care products (shower gel, body creams, etc.). Use natural facial care products. Use natural toothpaste. Use natural hair-care products such as shampoo, conditioner, gel, mousse, and hairspray. (For recommended products, visit www.BiblicalHealth Institute.com and click on the GPRx Resource Guide.)

Supplements: take one serving of a fiber/green superfood powder (mixed) or five caplets of a super green formula (swallowed with) twelve-to-sixteen ounces of water or raw vegetable juice (for recommended products, visit www.BiblicalHealthInstitute.com and click on the GPRx Resource Guide).

Body therapy: get twenty minutes of direct sunlight sometime during the day, but be careful between the hours of 10 a.m. to 2 p.m.

Exercise: perform functional fitness exercises for five to fifteen minutes or spend five to fifteen minutes on a mini trampoline. Finish with five to ten minutes of deep-breathing exercises. (One to three rounds of the exercises can be found at www.GreatPhysiciansRx.com.)

Emotional health: whenever you face a circumstance, such as your health, that causes you to worry, repeat the following: "Lord, I trust You. I cast my cares upon You, and I believe that You're going to take care of [insert your current situation] and make my health and make my body strong." Confess that throughout the day whenever you think about the condition of your health.

Breakfast

Make a smoothie in a blender with the following ingredients: 1 cup plain yogurt or kefir (goat's milk is best); 1 tablespoon organic flaxseed oil; 1 tablespoon organic raw honey; 1 cup organic fruit (berries, banana, peaches, pineapple, etc.); 2 tablespoons goat's milk protein powder (for recommended brands, visit www.BiblicalHealthInstitute.com and click on the GPRx Resource Guide); dash of vanilla extract (optional).

Supplements: take two whole food multivitamin caplets and one capsule of a whole food antioxidant/energy formula (for recommended brands, visit www.BiblicalHealthInstitute.com and click on the GPRx Resource Guide).

Lunch

Before eating, drink eight ounces of water.

During lunch, drink eight ounces of water or hot tea with honey.

large green salad with mixed greens, avocado, carrots, cucumbers, celery, tomatoes, red cabbage, red peppers, red onions, and sprouts with three hard-boiled omega-3 eggs

salad dressing: extra virgin olive oil, apple cider vinegar or lemon juice, Celtic Sea Salt, herbs, and spices, or mix one tablespoon of extra virgin olive oil with one tablespoon of a healthy store-bought dressing

one apple with skin

Supplements: take two whole food multivitamin caplets and one capsule of a whole food antioxidant/energy formula.

Dinner

Before eating, drink eight ounces of water.

During dinner, drink hot tea with honey (for recommended brands, visit www.BiblicalHealthInstitute.com and click on the GPRx Resource Guide).

baked, poached, or grilled wild-caught salmon

steamed broccoli

large green salad with mixed greens, avocado, carrots, cucumbers, celery, tomato, red cabbage, red onions, red peppers, and sprouts

salad dressing: extra virgin olive oil, apple cider vinegar or lemon juice, Celtic Sea Salt, herbs, and spices, or mix one tablespoon of extra virgin olive oil with one tablespoon of a healthy store-bought dressing

Supplements: take two whole food multivitamin caplets and one capsule of a whole food antioxidant blend and one-to-three teaspoons or three-to-nine capsules of a high omega-3 cod liver oil complex (for recommended brands, visit www.BiblicalHealthInstitute.com and click on the GPRx Resource Guide).

Snacks

apple slices with raw almond butter

one berry antioxidant whole food nutrition bar with beta-glucans from soluble oat fiber (for recommended brands, visit www.Biblical HealthInstitute.com and click on the GPRx Resource Guide).

Drink eight-to-twelve ounces of water, or hot or iced fresh-brewed tea with honey.

Before Bed

Exercise: go for a walk outdoors or participate in a favorite sport or recreational activity.

Supplements: take one serving of a fiber/green superfood powder (mixed) or five caplets of a super green formula (swallowed with) twelve-to-sixteen ounces of water or raw vegetable juice.

Body therapy: take a warm bath for fifteen minutes with eight drops of biblical essential oils added.

Advanced hygiene: repeat the advanced hygiene instructions from the morning of Day 1.

Emotional health: ask the Lord to bring to your mind someone you need to forgive. Take out a sheet of paper and write the person's name at the top. Try to remember each specific action that person did against you that brought you pain. Write down the following: "I forgive [insert person's name] for [insert the action he or she did against you]." After you fill up the paper, tear it up or burn it, and ask God to give you the strength to truly forgive that person.

Purpose: ask yourself these questions: "Did I live a life of purpose today?" "What did I do to add value to someone else's life today?" Commit to living a day of purpose tomorrow.

Prayer: thank God for this day, asking Him to give you a restoring night's rest and a fresh start tomorrow. Thank Him for His steadfast love that never ceases and His mercies new every morning. Read Romans 8:35, 37–39 out loud.

Sleep: go to bed by 10:30 p.m.

DAY 2

Upon Waking

Prayer: thank God because this is the day that the Lord has made. Rejoice and be glad in it. Thank Him for the breath in your lungs and the life in your body. Ask the Lord to heal your body and use your experience to benefit the lives of others. Read Psalm 91 out loud.

Purpose: ask the Lord to give you an opportunity to add significance to someone's life today. Watch for that opportunity. Ask God to use you this day for His intended purpose.

Advanced hygiene: follow the advanced hygiene recommendations from the morning of Day 1.

Reduce toxins: follow the recommendations to reduce toxins from the morning of Day 1.

Supplements: take one serving of a fiber/green superfood powder (mixed) or five caplets of a super green formula (swallowed with) twelve-to-sixteen ounces of water or raw vegetable juice.

Body therapy: take a hot and cold shower. After a normal shower, alternate sixty seconds of water as hot as you can stand it, followed by sixty seconds of water as cold as you can stand it. Repeat cycle four times for a total of eight minutes, finishing with cold.

Exercise: perform functional fitness exercises for five to fifteen minutes or spend five to fifteen minutes on a mini-trampoline. Finish with five to ten minutes of deep-breathing exercises. (One to three rounds of the exercises can be found at www.GreatPhysiciansRx.com.)

Emotional health: follow the emotional health recommendations from the morning of Day 1.

Breakfast

two or three eggs any style, cooked in one tablespoon of extra virgin coconut oil (for recommended brands, visit www.Biblical HealthInstitute.com and click on the GPRx Resource Guide)

stir-fried onions, mushrooms, and peppers

one slice of sprouted or yeast-free whole grain bread with almond butter and honey

Supplements: take two whole food multivitamin caplets and one capsule of a whole food antioxidant/energy formula.

Lunch

Before eating, drink eight ounces of water.

During lunch, drink eight ounces of water or hot tea with honey.

large green salad with mixed greens, avocado, carrots, tomato, red cabbage, red onions, red peppers, and sprouts with two ounces of low-mercury, high omega-3 tuna (for recommended brands, visit www.BiblicalHealthInstitute.com and click on the GPRx Resource Guide)

salad dressing: extra virgin olive oil, apple cider vinegar or lemon juice, Celtic Sea Salt, herbs, and spices, or mix one tablespoon of extra virgin olive oil with one tablespoon of a healthy store-bought dressing

organic grapes

Supplements: take two whole food multivitamin caplets and one capsule of a whole food antioxidant/energy formula.

Dinner

Before eating, drink eight ounces of water.

During dinner, drink hot tea with honey.

roasted organic chicken

cooked vegetables (carrots, onions, peas, etc.)

large green salad with mixed greens, avocado, carrots, tomato, red cabbage, red onions, red peppers, and sprouts

salad dressing: extra virgin olive oil, apple cider vinegar or lemon juice, Celtic Sea Salt, herbs, and spices, or mix one tablespoon of extra virgin olive oil with one tablespoon of a healthy store-bought dressing

Supplements: take two whole food multivitamin caplets and one capsule of a whole food antioxidant/energy blend and one to three teaspoons or three to nine capsules of a high omega-3 cod-liver oil complex.

Snacks

raw almonds and apple wedges

one chocolate protein whole food nutrition bar with beta-glucans from soluble oat fiber

Drink eight to twelve ounces of water, or hot or iced freshbrewed tea with honey.

Before Bed

Exercise: go for a walk outdoors or participate in a favorite sport or recreational activity.

Supplements: take one serving of a fiber/green superfood powder (mixed) or five caplets of a super green formula (swallowed with) twelve-to-sixteen ounces of water or raw vegetable juice.

Advanced hygiene: repeat the advanced hygiene instructions from the morning of Day 1.

Emotional health: repeat the emotional health recommendations from Day 1.

Purpose: ask yourself these questions: "Did I live a life of purpose today?" "What did I do to add value to someone else's life today?" Commit to living a day of purpose tomorrow.

Prayer: thank God for this day, asking Him to give you a restoring night's rest and a fresh start tomorrow. Thank Him for His steadfast love that never ceases and His mercies new every morning. Read 1 Corinthians 13:4–8 out loud.

Body therapy: spend ten minutes listening to soothing music before you retire.

Sleep: go to bed by 10:30 p.m.

Day 3

Upon Waking

Prayer: thank God because this is the day that the Lord has made. Rejoice and be glad in it. Thank Him for the breath in your lungs and the life in your body. Ask the Lord to heal your body and use your experience to benefit the lives of others. Read Ephesians 6:13–18 out loud.

Purpose: ask the Lord to give you an opportunity to add significance to someone's life today. Watch for that opportunity. Ask God to use you this day for His intended purpose.

Advanced hygiene: follow the advanced hygiene recommendations from the morning of Day 1.

Reduce toxins: follow the recommendations to reduce toxins from the morning of Day 1.

Supplements: take one serving of a fiber/green superfood powder (mixed) or five caplets of a super green formula (swallowed with) twelve-to-sixteen ounces of water or raw vegetable juice.

Body therapy: get twenty minutes of direct sunlight sometime during the day, but be careful between the hours of 10:00 a.m. and 2:00 p.m.

Exercise: perform functional fitness exercises for five to fifteen minutes or spend five to fifteen minutes on a mini-trampoline. Finish with five to ten minutes of deep-breathing exercises. (One to three rounds of the exercises can be found at www.GreatPhysiciansRx.com.)

Emotional health: follow the emotional health recommendations from Day 1.

Breakfast
four-to-eight ounces of organic whole milk yogurt or cottage cheese with fruit (pineapple, peaches or berries), honey, and a dash of vanilla extract

handful of raw almonds

one cup of hot tea with honey

Supplements: take two whole food multivitamin caplets and one capsule of a whole food antioxidant/energy formula.

Lunch
Before eating, drink eight ounces of water.

During lunch, drink eight ounces of water or hot tea with honey.

large green salad with mixed greens, avocado, carrots, cucumbers, celery, tomatoes, red cabbage, red peppers, red onions, and sprouts with three hard-boiled omega-3 eggs

salad dressing: extra virgin olive oil, apple cider vinegar or lemon juice, Celtic Sea Salt, herbs, and spices, or mix one tablespoon of extra virgin olive oil with one tablespoon of a healthy store-bought dressing

one piece of in-season fruit

Supplements: take two whole food multivitamin caplets and one capsule of a whole food antioxidant/energy formula.

Dinner
Before eating, drink eight ounces of water.

During dinner, drink hot tea with honey.

red meat steak (beef, buffalo, or venison)

steamed broccoli

baked sweet potato with butter

large green salad with mixed greens, avocado, carrots, cucumbers, celery, tomatoes, red cabbage, red peppers, red onions, and sprouts

salad dressing: extra virgin olive oil, apple cider vinegar or lemon juice, Celtic Sea Salt, herbs, and spices, or mix one tablespoon of extra virgin olive oil with one tablespoon of a healthy store-bought dressing

Supplements: take two whole food multivitamin caplets and one capsule of a whole food antioxidant/energy blend and one to three teaspoons or three to nine capsules of a high omega-3 cod-liver oil complex.

Snacks

four ounces of whole milk yogurt with fruit, honey, and a few almonds

one berry antioxidant whole food nutrition bar with beta-glucans from soluble oat fiber

Drink eight to twelve ounces of water, or hot or iced fresh-brewed tea with honey.

Before Bed

Exercise: go for a walk outdoors or participate in a favorite sport or recreational activity.

Supplements: take one serving of a fiber/green superfood powder (mixed) or five caplets of a super green formula (swallowed with) twelve-to-sixteen ounces of water or raw vegetable juice.

Body therapy: take a warm bath for fifteen minutes with eight drops of biblical essential oils added.

Advanced hygiene: follow the advanced hygiene instructions from the morning of Day 1.

Emotional health: follow the forgiveness recommendations from the evening of Day 1.

Purpose: ask yourself these questions: "Did I live a life of purpose today?" "What did I do to add value to someone else's life today?" Commit to living a day of purpose tomorrow.

Prayer: thank God for this day, asking Him to give you a restoring night's rest and a fresh start tomorrow. Thank Him for His steadfast love that never ceases and His mercies new every morning. Read Philippians 4:4–8, 11–13, 19 out loud.

Sleep: go to bed by 10:30 p.m.

Day 4

Upon Waking

Prayer: thank God because this is the day that the Lord has made. Rejoice and be glad in it. Thank Him for the breath in your lungs and the life in your body. Read Matthew 6:9–13 out loud.

Purpose: ask the Lord to give you an opportunity to add significance to someone's life today. Watch for that opportunity. Ask God to use you this day for His intended purpose.

Advanced hygiene: follow the advanced hygiene recommendations from Day 1.

Reduce toxins: follow the recommendations for reducing toxins from Day 1.

Supplements: take one serving of a fiber/green superfood powder (mixed) or five caplets of a super green formula (swallowed with) twelve-to-sixteen ounces of water or raw vegetable juice.

Exercise: perform functional fitness exercises for five to fifteen minutes or spend five to fifteen minutes on a mini-trampoline. Finish with five to ten minutes of deep-breathing exercises. (One to three rounds of the exercises can be found at www.GreatPhysiciansRx.com.)

Body therapy: take a hot and cold shower. After a normal shower, alternate sixty seconds of water as hot as you can stand it, followed by sixty seconds of water as cold as you can stand it. Repeat cycle four times for a total of eight minutes, finishing with cold.

Emotional health: follow the emotional health recommendations from the morning of Day 1.

Breakfast

three soft-boiled or poached eggs

four ounces of sprouted whole grain cereal with two ounces of whole milk yogurt or goat's milk (for recommended brands, visit www.BiblicalHealthInstitute.com and click on the GPRx Resource Guide)

one cup of hot tea with honey

Supplements: take two whole food multivitamin caplets and one capsule of a whole food antioxidant/energy formula.

Lunch

Before eating, drink eight ounces of water.

During lunch, drink eight ounces of water or hot tea with honey.

large green salad with mixed greens, avocado, carrots, cucumbers, celery, tomatoes, red cabbage, red peppers, red onions, and sprouts with three ounces of canned tuna

salad dressing: extra virgin olive oil, apple cider vinegar or lemon juice, Celtic Sea Salt, herbs, and spices, or mix one tablespoon of extra virgin olive oil with one tablespoon of a healthy store-bought dressing one bunch of grapes with seeds

Supplements: take two whole food multivitamin caplets and one capsule of a whole food antioxidant/energy formula.

Dinner

Before eating, drink eight ounces of water.

During dinner, drink hot tea with honey.

grilled chicken breast

steamed veggies

small portion of cooked whole grain (quinoa, amaranth, millet, or brown rice) cooked with one tablespoon of extra virgin coconut oil

large green salad with mixed greens, avocado, carrots, cucumbers, celery, tomatoes, red cabbage, red peppers, red onions, and sprouts

salad dressing: extra virgin olive oil, apple cider vinegar or lemon juice, Celtic Sea Salt, herbs, and spices, or mix one tablespoon of extra virgin olive oil with one tablespoon of a healthy store-bought dressing

Supplements: take two whole food multivitamin caplets and two capsules of a whole food antioxidant blend and one to three teaspoons or three to nine capsules of a high omega-3 cod-liver oil complex.

Snacks

apple and carrots with raw almond butter

one berry antioxidant whole food nutrition bar with beta-glucans from soluble oat fiber

Drink eight to twelve ounces of water, or hot or iced fresh-brewed tea with honey.

Before Bed

Drink eight to twelve ounces of water or hot tea with honey.

Exercise: go for a walk outdoors or participate in a favorite sport or recreational activity.

Supplements: take one serving of a fiber/green superfood powder (mixed) or five caplets of a super green formula (swallowed with) twelve-to-sixteen ounces of water or raw vegetable juice.

Advanced hygiene: follow the advanced hygiene recommendations from the morning of Day 1.

Emotional health: follow the forgiveness recommendations from the evening of Day 1.

Purpose: ask yourself these questions: "Did I live a life of purpose today?" "What did I do to add value to someone else's life today?" Commit to living a day of purpose tomorrow.

Prayer: thank God for this day, asking Him to give you a restoring night's rest and a fresh start tomorrow. Thank Him for His steadfast love that never ceases and His mercies that are new every morning. Read Romans 8:35, 37–39 out loud.

Body therapy: spend ten minutes listening to soothing music before you retire.

Sleep: go to bed by 10:30 p.m.

Day 5 (Partial Fast Day)

Upon Waking

Prayer: thank God because this is the day that the Lord has made. Rejoice and be glad in it. Thank Him for the breath in your lungs and the life in your body. Read Isaiah 58:6–9 out loud.

Purpose: ask the Lord to give you an opportunity to add significance to someone's life today. Watch for that opportunity. Ask God to use you this day for His intended purpose.

Advanced hygiene: follow the advanced hygiene recommendations from Day 1.

Reduce toxins: follow the recommendations for reducing toxins from Day 1.

Supplements: take one serving of a fiber/green superfood powder (mixed) or five caplets of a super green formula (swallowed with) twelve-to-sixteen ounces of water or raw vegetable juice.

Exercise: perform functional fitness exercises for five to fifteen minutes or spend five to fifteen minutes on a mini-trampoline. Finish with five to ten minutes of deep-breathing exercises.

Body therapy: get twenty minutes of direct sunlight sometime during the day, but be careful between the hours of 10:00 a.m. and 2:00 p.m.

Emotional health: follow the emotional health recommendations from the morning of Day 1.

Breakfast
none (partial fast day)

eight to twelve ounces of water

Supplements: take two whole food multivitamin caplets and one capsule of a whole food antioxidant/energy formula.

Lunch
none (partial fast day)

Supplements: take two whole food multivitamin caplets and one capsule of a whole food antioxidant/energy formula.

Dinner

Before eating, drink eight ounces of water.

During dinner, drink hot tea with honey.

chicken soup (visit www.BiblicalHealthInstitute.com for the recipe)

cultured vegetables (for recommended brands, visit www.Biblical HealthInstitute.com and click on the GPRx Resource Guide)

large green salad with mixed greens, avocado, carrots, cucumbers, celery, tomatoes, red cabbage, red peppers, red onions, and sprouts

salad dressing: extra virgin olive oil, apple cider vinegar or lemon juice, Celtic Sea Salt, herbs, and spices, or mix one tablespoon of extra virgin olive oil with one tablespoon of a healthy store-bought dressing

Supplements: take two whole food multivitamin caplets and two capsules of a whole food antioxidant blend and one to three teaspoons or three to nine capsules of a high omega-3 cod-liver oil complex.

Snacks

none (partial fast day)

drink eight ounces of water

Before Bed

Drink eight to twelve ounces of water or hot tea with honey.

Exercise: go for a walk outdoors or participate in a favorite sport or recreational activity.

Supplements: take one serving of a fiber/green superfood powder (mixed) or five caplets of a super green formula (swallowed with) twelve-to-sixteen ounces of water or raw vegetable juice.

Advanced hygiene: follow the advanced hygiene recommendations from the morning of Day 1.

Emotional health: follow the forgiveness recommendations from the evening of Day 1.

Body therapy: take a warm bath for fifteen minutes with eight drops of biblical essential oils added.

Purpose: ask yourself these questions: "Did I live a life of purpose today?" "What did I do to add value to someone else's life today?" Commit to living a day of purpose tomorrow.

Prayer: thank God for this day, asking Him to give you a restoring night's rest and a fresh start tomorrow. Thank Him for His steadfast love that never ceases and His mercies that are new every morning. Read Isaiah 58:6–9 out loud.

Sleep: go to bed by 10:30 p.m.

DAY 6 (REST DAY)

Upon Waking

Prayer: thank God because this is the day that the Lord has made. Rejoice and be glad in it. Thank Him for the breath in your lungs and the life in your body. Read Psalm 23 out loud.

Purpose: ask the Lord to give you an opportunity to add significance to someone's life today. Watch for that opportunity. Ask God to use you this day for His intended purpose.

Advanced hygiene: follow the advanced hygiene recommendations from Day 1.

Reduce toxins: follow the recommendations for reducing toxins from Day 1.

Supplements: take one serving of a fiber/green superfood powder (mixed) or five caplets of a super green formula (swallowed with) twelve-to-sixteen ounces of water or raw vegetable juice.

Exercise: no formal exercise since it's a rest day.

Body therapies: none since it's a rest day.

Emotional health: follow the emotional health recommendations from the morning of Day 1.

Breakfast

two or three eggs cooked any style in one tablespoon of extra virgin coconut oil

one grapefruit or orange

handful of almonds

Supplements: take two whole food multivitamin caplets and one capsule of a whole food antioxidant/energy formula.

Lunch

Before eating, drink eight ounces of water.

During lunch, drink eight ounces of water or hot tea with honey.

large green salad with mixed greens, avocado, carrots, cucumbers, celery, tomatoes, red cabbage, red peppers, red onions, and sprouts with two ounces of low-mercury, high omega-3 tuna.

salad dressing: extra virgin olive oil, apple cider vinegar or lemon juice, Celtic Sea Salt, herbs, and spices, or mix one tablespoon of extra virgin olive oil with one tablespoon of a healthy store-bought dressing

one organic apple with the skin

Supplements: take two whole food multivitamin caplets and one capsule of a whole food antioxidant/energy formula.

Dinner

Before eating, drink eight ounces of water.

During dinner, drink hot tea with honey.

roasted organic chicken

cooked vegetables (carrots, onions, peas, etc.)

large green salad with mixed greens, carrots, cucumbers, celery, tomatoes, red cabbage, red peppers, red onions, and sprouts

salad dressing: extra virgin olive oil, apple cider vinegar or lemon juice, Celtic Sea Salt, herbs, and spices, or mix one tablespoon of extra virgin olive oil with one tablespoon of a healthy store-bought dressing

Supplements: take two whole food multivitamin caplets and two capsules of a whole food antioxidant/energy blend and one to three teaspoons or three to nine capsules of a high omega-3 cod-liver oil complex.

Snacks

handful of raw almonds with apple wedges

one berry antioxidant whole food nutrition bar with beta-glucans from soluble oat fiber

Drink eight to twelve ounces of water, or hot or iced fresh-brewed tea with honey.

Before Bed

Drink eight to twelve ounces of water or hot tea with honey.

Exercise: go for a walk outdoors or participate in a favorite sport or recreational activity.

Supplements: take one serving of a fiber/green superfood powder (mixed) or five caplets of a super green formula (swallowed with) twelve-to-sixteen ounces of water or raw vegetable juice.

Advanced hygiene: follow the advanced hygiene recommendations from the morning of Day 1.

Emotional health: follow the forgiveness recommendations from the evening of Day 1.

Purpose: ask yourself these questions: "Did I live a life of purpose today?" "What did I do to add value to someone else's life today?" Commit to living a day of purpose tomorrow.

Prayer: thank God for this day, asking Him to give you a restoring night's rest and a fresh start tomorrow. Thank Him for His steadfast love that never ceases and His mercies that are new every morning. Read Psalm 23 out loud.

Body therapy: spend ten minutes listening to soothing music before you retire.

Sleep: go to bed by 10:30 p.m.

DAY 7

Upon Waking

Prayer: thank God because this is the day that the Lord has made. Rejoice and be glad in it. Thank Him for the breath in your lungs and the life in your body. Read Psalm 91 out loud.

Purpose: ask the Lord to give you an opportunity to add significance to someone's life today. Watch for that opportunity. Ask God to use you this day for His intended purpose.

Advanced hygiene: follow the advanced hygiene recommendations from Day 1.

Reduce toxins: follow the recommendations for reducing toxins from Day 1.

Supplements: take one serving of a fiber/green superfood powder (mixed) or five caplets of a super green formula (swallowed with) twelve-to-sixteen ounces of water or raw vegetable juice.

Exercise: perform functional fitness exercises for five to fifteen minutes or spend five to fifteen minutes on a mini-trampoline. Finish with five to ten minutes of deep-breathing exercises.

Body therapy: get twenty minutes of direct sunlight sometime during the day, but be careful between the hours of 10:00 a.m. and 2:00 p.m.

Emotional health: follow the emotional health recommendations from the morning of Day 1.

Breakfast

Make a smoothie in a blender with the following ingredients: 1 cup plain yogurt or kefir (goat's milk is best); 1 tablespoon organic flaxseed oil; 1 tablespoon organic raw honey; 1 cup organic fruit (berries, banana, peaches, pineapple, etc.); 2 tablespoons goat's milk protein powder; dash of vanilla extract (optional).

Supplements: take two whole food multivitamin caplets and one capsule of a whole food antioxidant/energy formula.

Lunch

Before eating, drink eight ounces of water.

During lunch, drink eight ounces of water or hot tea with honey.

large green salad with mixed greens, raw goat cheese, avocado, carrots, cucumbers, celery, tomatoes, red cabbage, red peppers, red onions, and sprouts with three ounces of cold, poached, or canned wild-caught salmon

salad dressing: extra virgin olive oil, apple cider vinegar or lemon juice, Celtic Sea Salt, herbs, and spices, or mix one tablespoon of extra virgin olive oil with one tablespoon of a healthy store-bought dressing

one piece of in-season fruit

Supplements: take two whole food multivitamin caplets and one capsule of a whole food antioxidant/energy formula.

Dinner

Before eating, drink eight ounces of water.

During dinner, drink hot tea with honey.

baked or grilled fish of your choice

steamed broccoli

baked sweet potato with butter

large green salad with mixed greens, carrots, cucumbers, celery, tomatoes, red cabbage, red peppers, red onions, and sprouts

salad dressing: extra virgin olive oil, apple cider vinegar or lemon juice, Celtic Sea Salt, herbs, and spices, or mix one tablespoon of extra virgin olive oil with one tablespoon of a healthy store-bought dressing

Supplements: take two whole food multivitamin caplets and one capsule of a whole food antioxidant/energy blend and one to three teaspoons or three to nine capsules of a high omega-3 cod-liver oil complex.

Snacks

apple slices with raw sesame butter (tahini)

one berry antioxidant whole food nutrition bar with beta-glucans from soluble oat fiber

Drink eight to twelve ounces of water, or hot or iced fresh-brewed tea with honey.

Before Bed

Drink eight to twelve ounces of water or hot tea with honey.

Exercise: go for a walk outdoors or participate in a favorite sport or recreational activity.

Supplements: take one serving of a fiber/green superfood powder (mixed) or five caplets of a super green formula (swallowed with) twelve-to-sixteen ounces of water or raw vegetable juice.

Advanced hygiene: follow the advanced hygiene recommendations from the morning of Day 1.

Emotional health: follow the forgiveness recommendations from the evening of Day 1.

Body therapy: take a warm bath for fifteen minutes with eight drops of biblical essential oils added.

Purpose: ask yourself these questions: "Did I live a life of purpose today?" "What did I do to add value to someone else's life today?" Commit to living a day of purpose tomorrow.

Prayer: thank God for this day, asking Him to give you a restoring night's rest and a fresh start tomorrow. Thank Him for His steadfast love that never ceases and His mercies that are new every morning. Read 1 Corinthians 13:4–8 out loud.

Sleep: go to bed by 10:30 p.m.

DAY 8 AND BEYOND

If you're feeling better, you can repeat the Great Physician's Rx for a Healthy Heart Battle Plan as many times as you'd like. For detailed step-by-step suggestions and meal and lifestyle plans, visit www.GreatPhysiciansRx.com and join the 40-Day Health Experience for continued good health. Or, if you want to maintain your newfound level of health, you may be interested in the Lifetime of Wellness plan. These online programs will provide you with customized daily meal-and-exercise plans and the tools to track your progress.

If you've experienced positive results from the Great Physician's Rx for a Healthy Heart program, I encourage you to reach out to someone you know and recommend this book and program to them. You can learn how to lead a small group at your church or home by visiting www.GreatPhysiciansRx.com.

Remember: You don't have to be a doctor or a health expert to help transform the life of someone you care about—you just have to be willing.

Allow me to offer you this prayer of blessing paraphrased from Numbers 6:24–26:

May the Lord bless you and keep you.
May the Lord make His face to shine upon you and be
    gracious unto you.
May the Lord lift up His countenance upon you and bring you
    peace.
In the name of Yeshua Ha Mashiach, Jesus our Messiah.
Amen.

Need Recipes?

For a detailed list of over two hundred healthy and delicious recipes contained in the Great Physician's Rx eating plan, please visit www.BiblicalHealthInstitute.com.

NOTES

Introduction

1. "Cardiovascular Statistics Updated for 2005," from the American Heart Association's year-end report, December 30, 2004.

2. "Heart Disease and Stroke Statistics—2006 Update," from the online magazine *Circulation*, published by the American Heart Association, January 11, 2006, and available at http://www.circulationaha.org.

3. Ibid.

4. "The Heart Truth for Women," a press release issued by the National Heart, Lung, and Blood Institute, part of the National Institutes of Health. "The Heart Truth" is a national awareness campaign for women about heart disease and can be viewed online at www.nhlbi.nih.gov/health/hearttruth.

5. "Marketing an Operation: Coronary Artery Bypass Surgery," a paper by Thomas A. Preston, MD, associated with the Mount Rainer Clinic and available at www.drcranton.com/chelation/cabg1.htm.

6. From "Oral EDTA Helps Restore Cardiovascular Function," by Dr. Gail Valentine, and available on the Life Enhancement Web site at www.life-enhancement.com/article_template.asp?ID=531.

7. "Chelation Therapy: AHA Recommendation," found on the American Heart Association Web site at www.americanheart.org/presenter.jhtml?identifier=4493.

8. American Heart Association's *Congenital Heart Defects Report*, July 8, 2005.

Key #1

1. The Framingham Heart Study, under the direction of the National Heart, Lung, and Blood Institute, can be viewed at http://www.nhlbi.nih.gov/about/Framingham/.

2. Alex Berenson, "Lipitor or Generic? Billion-Dollar Battle Looms," *New York Times*, 15 October, 2005.

3. K. M. Anderson, W. P. Castelli, and D. Levy, "Cholesterol and mortality. 30 years of follow-up from the Framingham study," *JAMA* 257, 2176-80 (1987).

4. Sue Goetinck, "Researchers Cite Protein in Heart Protection," *Dallas Morning News*, 24 November 2005.

5. *FDA Consumer* magazine, July-August 1997 issue, publication number (FDA) 97-2313.

6. *American Journal of Clinical Nutrition,* December 2004, vol 80:1492–9 and available at www.wholegrainscouncil.org/research.htm.

7. "Fiber May Reduce Women's Risk of Heart Disease," posted July 1, 1999, on www.cnn.com.

8. "Dietary Supplement Fact Sheet: Vitamin B-12," from the Office of Dietary Supplement, National Institute of Health Clinical Center, and available at www.ods.od.nih.gov/factsheets/vitaminb12.asp#h9.

9. "Omega-3 Fatty Acids" article available at www.wholehealthmd.com/refshelf/substances_view/1,1525,992,00.html.

10. "Fats and Cholesterol," found on the Harvard School of Public Health and available at www.hsph.harvard.edu/nutritionsource/fats.html.

11. "Oxygenated Carotenoid Lutein and Progression of Early Atherosclerosis: The Los Angeles Atherosclerosis Study, James H. Dwyer, PhD, Mohamad Navab, PhD, Kathleen M. Dwyer, PhD, et. al, American Heart Association *Circulation* magazine, 2001;103:2922, and available at www.circ.ahajournals.org/cgi/content/abstract/103/24/2922.

12. From "Fruits and Vegetables," published by the Harvard School of Public Health, December 13, 2004, and available at www.hsph.harvard.edu/nutritionsource.

13. Steven Milloy, Fox News reporter, "Healthy Food Labeling: Buyer Beware," July 18, 2003, available at http://www.foxnews.com/story/0,2933,92249,00.html.

14. "Nuts Cut Coronary Heart Disease Risk," a May 8, 2001, press release by Penn State University and available at http://www.psu.edu/ur/2001/nuts.html.

15. Paul Schulick, *Ginger: Common Spice & Wonder Drug,* Third Edition (Prescott, AZ: Hohm Press, 1996), 36.

16. "Loma Linda University Reveals First Study on Correlation between High Water Intake and Lowered Coronary Heart Disease," a press release issued April 25, 2002, and available at www.llu.edu/news/pr/042502water.html.

17. F. Batmanghelidj, MD, *You're Not Sick, You're Thirsty!* (New York: Warner Books), 206.

Key #3
1. Christine Gorman and Alic Park, "Inflammation Is a Secret Killer: The Surprising Link Between Inflammation and Asthma, Heart Attacks, Cancer, Alzheimer's and Other Diseases," *Time*, 23 February 2004.

2. "Heart Disease and Stroke," an article found on the American Academy of Periodontology Web site and available at www.perio.org/consumer/mbc.heart.htm.

Key #5
1. From two press reports: "Bad Air Causes Heart Disease, Says U.S. Group," by Reuters News Agency, June 3, 2004, and "Air Pollution, Even at 'Safe Levels,' Is Bad for the Heart," by the American Heart Association, November 11, 2003.

Key #6
1. Joel Achenbach, *Why Things Are: Answers to Every Essential Question in Life* (New York: Ballantine Books, 1991).

2. Don Colbert, MD, *Deadly Emotions: Understanding the Mind-Body-Spirit Connection That Can Heal or Destroy You* (Nashville: Nelson Publishers, 2003), 38-39.

Key #7
1. Germain Copeland, *Prayers That Avail Much* (Tulsa: Harrison House, 1997), 104–105.

2. Hilary E. MacGregor, "Researchers Look at the Power of Prayer," *Los Angeles Times*, 1 June 2005.

ABOUT THE AUTHORS

Jordan Rubin has dedicated his life to transforming the health of others one life at a time. He is a certified nutritional consultant, a certified personal fitness instructor, a certified nutrition specialist, and a member of the National Academy of Sports Medicine.

Mr. Rubin is the founder and chairman of Garden of Life, Inc., a health and wellness company based in West Palm Beach, Florida, that produces whole food nutritional supplements and personal care products. He is also president and CEO of GPRx, Inc., a biblically based health and wellness company providing educational resources, small group curriculum, functional foods, nutritional supplements, and wellness services.

He and his wife, Nicki, married in 1999 and are the parents of a toddler-aged son, Joshua. They make their home in Palm Beach Gardens, Florida.

Joseph D. Brasco, M.D., has extensive knowledge and experience in gastroenterology and internal medicine. He attended medical school at Medical College of Wisconsin in Milwaukee, Wisconsin, and is board certified with the American Board of Internal Medicine. Besides writing for various medical journals, he is also the coauthor of *Restoring Your Digestive Health* with Jordan Rubin.

BHI

BIBLICAL HEALTH
INSTITUTE

The Biblical Health Institute (www.BiblicalHealthInstitute.com) is an online learning community housing educational resources and curricula reinforcing and expanding on Jordan Rubin's Biblical Health message.

Biblical Health Institute provides:

1. "101" level **FREE**, introductory courses corresponding to Jordan's book The Great Physician's Rx for Health and Wellness and its seven keys; Current "101" courses include:

   * "Eating to Live 101"

   * "Whole Food Nutrition Supplements 101"

   * "Advanced Hygiene 101"

   * "Exercise and Body Therapies 101"

   * "Reducing Toxins 101"

   * "Emotional Health 101"

   * "Prayer and Purpose 101"

2. **FREE** resources (healthy recipes, what to E.A.T., resource guide)

3. **FREE** media--videos and video clips of Jordan, music therapy samples, etc.--and much more!

Additionally, Biblical Health Institute also offers in-depth courses for those who want to go deeper.

Course offerings include:

   * 40-hour certificate program to become a Biblical Health Coach

   * A la carte course offerings designed for personal study and growth (launching late April 2006)

   * Home school courses developed by Christian educators, supporting home-schooled students and their parents (designed for middle school and high school ages—launching in August 2006).

For more information and updates on these and other resources go to
www.BiblicalHealthInstitute.com

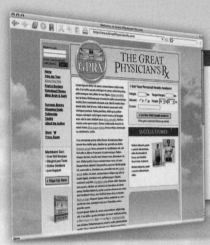

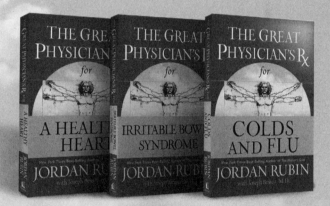

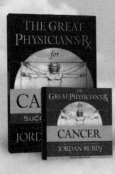 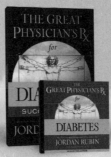 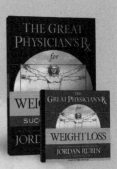